EARLY BREAST CANCER

EARLY BREAST CANCER

Detection and Treatment

EDITED BY

H. STEPHEN GALLAGER, M.D.
The University of Texas M. D. Anderson Hospital and Tumor Institute

CONFERENCE SPONSORED BY
American College of Radiology
The American Cancer Society
Cancer Control Program of the National Cancer Institute

A WILEY BIOMEDICAL PUBLICATION

JOHN WILEY & SONS, New York ● London ● Sydney ● Toronto

Published by John Wiley & Sons, Inc.
All rights reserved. Published simultaneously in Canada.

Library of Congress Cataloging in Publication Data:
Conference on Detection and Treatment of Early
        Breast Cancer, 13th, Lake Buena Vista, Fla.,
        1974.
        Early breast cancer.

        "A Wiley biomedical publication."
        Conference arranged by the Committee on Mammog-
raphy and Diseases of the Breast, American College
of Radiology.
        Bibliography: p.
        Includes index.
        1. Breast—Cancer—Diagnosis—Congresses.
2. Cancer—Prevention—Congresses. 3. Breast—
Cancer—Surgery—Congresses. I. Gallager, H.
Stephen, 1922-   II. American College of Radiology. Committee on Mammography and Diseases of the
Breast. III. Title. [DNLM: 1. Breast neoplasms—Diagnosis—Congresses. 2. Breast neoplasms—Prevention and control—Congresses. 3. Mammography—Congresses. WP870 C215]
RC280.B8C63 1974   616.9'94'49   75-23327
ISBN 0-471-29061-0

Printed in the United States of America

10 9 8 7 6 5 4 3 2 1

Contributors

Franklin S. Alcorn, M.D., Attending Radiologist, Presbyterian–St. Luke's Hospital and Professor of Radiology, Rush Medical College, Chicago.

David E. Anderson, Ph.D., Professor of Biology, The University of Texas M. D. Anderson Hospital and Tumor Institute, Houston.

Donald E. Bauermeister, M.D., Department of Pathology, Virginia Mason Medical Center, Seattle.

Benjamin F. Byrd, Jr., M.D., Clinical Professor of Surgery, Vanderbilt University School of Medicine and Meharry Medical School, Nashville.

Thomas Carlile, M.D., Department of Radiology, The Mason Clinic, Seattle.

James T. De Luca, M.D., Chief of Radiology, The Community Hospital at Glen Cove, New York.

Gerald D. Dodd, M.D., Professor Diagnostic Radiology, The University of Texas M. D. Anderson Hospital and Tumor Institute, Houston.

Alan S. Baker, M.S., Medical Physicist, Division of Radiology, Albert Einstein Medical Center, Philadelphia.

Robert L. Egan, M.D., Chief, Section of Mammography, Emory University School of Medicine, Atlanta.

Bernard Fisher, M.D., Professor of Surgery, University of Pittsburgh School of Medicine, Pittsburgh.

H. Stephen Gallager, M.D., Associate Pathologist, The University of Texas M. D. Anderson Hospital and Tumor Institute, Houston.

Richard H. Gold, M.D., Assistant Professor of Radiological Sciences, and

Chief, Section of Mammography, UCLA Center for the Health Sciences, Los Angeles.

Laman A. Gray, M.D., Clinical Professor of Obstetrics and Gynecology, University of Louisville School of Medicine, Louisville.

E. Cuyler Hammond, Sc.D., Vice President, Epidemiology and Statistics, American Cancer Society, Inc., New York.

William G. Hammond, M.D., Chief, Clinical Investigations Branch, National Cancer Institute, Washington.

Charles W. Hayden, M.D., Consultant in Surgery, The Community Hospital at Glen Cove, New York.

Arthur I. Holleb, M.D., Senior Vice President for Medical Affairs and Research, American Cancer Society, Inc., New York.

Robert V. P. Hutter, M.D., Director, Anatomic Pathology, St. Barnabas Medical Center, Livingston, New Jersey.

Harold J. Isard, M.D., Chairman, Division of Radiology, Albert Einstein Medical Center, Philadelphia.

Roberta L. A. Kirch, M.D., Department of Radiology, Memorial Hospital for Cancer and Allied Diseases, New York.

Henry P. Leis, Jr., M.D., Clinical Professor of Surgery, and Chief, Breast Service, New York Medical College, New York.

Richard G. Lester, M.D., Professor and Chairman, Radiology, Duke University Medical School, Durham.

William M. Markel, M.D., Vice President for Service and Rehabilitation, American Cancer Society, Inc., New York.

John E. Martin, M.D., Head, Department of Radiology, St. Joseph Hospital, Houston.

Marvin V. McClow, M.D., Director, Department of Radiology, St. Vincent's Hospital, Jacksonville.

Condict Moore, M.D., Professor of Surgery (Oncology), University of Louisville School of Medicine, Louisville.

Eleanor D. Montague, M.D., Radiotherapist and Professor of Radiotherapy, The University of Texas M.D. Anderson Hospital and Tumor Institute, Houston.

David D. Paulus, M.D., Associate Radiologist, The University of Texas M. D. Anderson Hospital and Tumor Institute, Houston.

R. Waldo Powell, M.D., Associate Professor of Surgery, Emory University Clinic and Emory University School of Medicine, Atlanta.

William E. Powers, M.D., Professor of Radiology and Director, Division of Radiation Oncology, Washington University School of Medicine, St. Louis.

Robert W. Roberston, Jr., M.S., Senior Medical Student, University of Louisville School of Medicine, Louisville.

Guy F. Robbins, M.D., Acting Chief, Breast Service, and Director of Rehabilitation Program, Memorial Hospital for Cancer and Allied Diseases, New York.

George P. Rosemond, M.D., Professor of Surgery, Temple University School of Medicine, Philadelphia.

Paul Peter Rosen, M.D., Associate Attending Pathologist, Memorial Hospital for Cancer and Allied Diseases, New York.

Sam Shapiro, Director, Health Services Research and Development Center, Johns Hopkins Medical Institutions, and Professor of Medical Care and Hospitals, School of Hygiene and Public Health, Johns Hopkins University, Baltimore.

William W. Shingleton, M.D., Professor of Surgery, and Chief, Division of General Surgery, Duke University Medical Center, Durham.

Ruth E. Snyder, M.D., Associate Radiologist, Memorial Hospital for Cancer and Allied Diseases, and Clinical Assistant Professor of Radiology, Cornell University Medical School, New York.

Reuven K. Snyderman, M.D., Chief, Division of Plastic Surgery, Raritan Valley Hospital, and Clinical Associate Professor of Surgery (Plastic), Rutgers Medical School, Princeton.

Justin J. Stein, M.D., Professor of Radiological Sciences (Radiation Therapy), UCLA Center for Health Sciences and President, American Cancer Society, Inc., Los Angeles.

Philip Strax, M.D. Medical Director, Guttman Institute, New York.

Herbert B. Taylor, M.D., Professor of Pathology, St. Louis University School of Medicine, St. Louis.

Willis J. Taylor, M.D., Department of Radiology, The Mason Clinic, Seattle.

Jerome A. Urban, M.D., Attending Surgeon, Memorial-Sloan-Kettering Cancer Center, and Associate Clinical Professor of Surgery, Cornell University Medical Center, New York.

Louis Venet, M.D., Associate Director, Department of Surgery, Beth Israel Medical Center, and Associate Clinical Professor of Surgery, Mt. Sinai School of Medicine, New York.

Wanda Venet, R.N., Director of Operations, Breast Cancer Screening Program, Health Insurance Plan of Greater New York, New York.

J. D. Wallace,* Research Professor Radiology, Thomas Jefferson University, Philadelphia.

*deceased

Ashbel C. Williams, M.D., Surgeon, St. Vincent's Hospital, Jacksonville.

David A. Wood, M.D., Director Emeritus, Cancer Research Institute, and Professor of Pathology Emeritus, University of California, San Francisco.

Alfonso Zermeno, Ph.D., Head, Section of Experimental Diagnostic Radiology, The University of Texas M. D. Anderson Hospital and Tumor Institute, Houston.

Foreword

Although everyone greatly respected his stature in the world of medicine, Wendell G. Scott was the kind of man one naturally called "Scottie," and I shall continue to do so herein. Scottie was a radiologist of eminence, a teacher, an author, an editor, a husband, a father, and a leader of men. To any task in his rich and variegated life, he characteristically brought a dynamic and forceful spirit of great influence. Some of Scottie's philosophy was summed up in his 1964 presidential address to the American Cancer Society:

> The onrushing flood of future possibilities brings with it a spirit of adventure; a need for bold, imaginative thinking, a willingness to gamble on provocative new concepts; the courage to break away from entrenched viewpoints, and the aggressiveness to bring this into reality.

Twenty-five years ago or so, Scottie's leadership contributed to the amalgamation of the St. Louis Division of the American Cancer Society and the Missouri Division, thus strengthening both. In rapid succession, Scottie became a director of the American Cancer Society, chairman of its Medical and Scientific Committee, President (1963-64), Honorary Life Member of its Board of Directors, and recipient of the Annual National Award. He received these last two honors, representing the Society's highest citations for achievement, in 1971.

Of added interest were Scottie's concomitant activities in the Cancer Program of the Federal Government. In the early 1960s, Scottie became a member of the Cancer Control Advisory Committee, of which Dr. Lewis C. Robbins and I were then cochairmen. I well remember the decision to initiate a nationwide program in mammography. First, the Cancer Control program gave support to the development of a training program for professional and paramedical personnel at M. D. Anderson Hospital and Tumor Institute under Dr. Robert Egan's direction. Subsequently, Dr. John Paul Lindsay and others of the Advisory Committee visited various schools of medicine to ascertain their interest and to encourage their participation in a nationwide mammography training program. The first Conference on Mammography and Diseases of the Breast was held in Houston in 1960 with Dr. Egan as chairman and possibly 20 radiologists in attendance.

In this earlier Cancer Control Program, then under the Bureau of State Services, Scottie also lent his enthusiastic support to the launching of a program of senior clinical cancer traineeships. These were planned to provide special knowledge of cancer for young physicians in the specialties of radiation therapy, diagnostic radiology, pathology, surgery, and internal medicine. The rest of the story of mammography and traineeships is well known to everyone and needs no elaboration.

Dr. Scott promoted cancer education at all levels, including his editorship of the journal *Cancer*. He also looked beyond the problems of management of the patient with cancer. In the 1969 L. Henry Garland Memorial Lecture, presented at the ninety-eighth Annual Meeting of the California Medical Association, he chose as his topic "New Concepts in Cancer Control —Preventable and Avoidable Cancer." In this he directed attention to prevention, a challenge even greater than that of early diagnosis, treatment, and rehabilitation. Agreeing with the remarks of Sir Alexander Haddow at the Ninth International Cancer Congress that "the majority of human cancers are avoidable," Dr. Scott concluded the Garland lecture with the following words:

> While we are awaiting the final solution of the cancer enigma that will come from further basic research, great efforts are justified for the full development of programs on avoidable and preventable cancers and those arising from personal indifference. For the past two decades the great emphasis has been on furthering cancer research, and rightly so. The time has now come to direct emphasis to the prevention and avoidance of cancer and to teach people that cancers can arise from self-neglect.

Ever ready to assist the national effort in its war on cancer, Scottie gave unstintingly of his time to congressional hearings and to the efforts that culminated in enactment of the National Cancer Act of 1971. Later, he was chosen to serve as one of the first members of the enlarged and reconstituted National Advisory Cancer Board.

Scottie's commitment to the nation was exemplified by his service during World War II. He later continued in the active reserve as Consultant to the Surgeon General and retired with the well-deserved rank of Rear Admiral.

As a firm believer in voluntarism, Scottie served as a member of the Council on Voluntary Health Agencies of the American Medical Association.

Scottie was a Chancellor of the American College of Radiology and a liaison member of the Cancer Commission of the American College of Surgeons. In this latter role he was a key member from 1967 through 1971 of the "Cole Committee" on Guidelines for Care of the Cancer Patient and was author of the chapter on diagnostic radiology in its report published in January 1971.

The wide scope of activities and the significant accomplishments of this exceptional man were made possible in no small degree by the intense interest and devoted support of his constant partner and wife, Ella. She rarely failed to accompany him to meetings such as mammography conferences, the meetings of the American Cancer Society, and the annual meetings of the American College of Radiology. Today she carries forward the torch of many activities that were close to Scottie.

Establishment by Washington University of the Wendell G. Scott Lectureship Fund in the spring of 1972 was an honor Scottie cherished highly. With much anticipation he looked forward to attendance at the May 18 dinner at which the Lectureship was to be formally announced and his portrait by Fred Conway unveiled. Fate decreed otherwise. His career was terminated cruelly by cancer on May 3, 1972.

Wendell G. Scott contributed much to the welfare and health of the people of the United States and played a leading role in advancing cancer education and in supporting research and cancer control. Because of his dedicated efforts on behalf of the development of mammography, it is appropriate that this volume is dedicated to him.

DAVID A. WOOD, M.D.

Introduction

The first of these annual conferences on breast cancer was held in 1961 and although 13 years does not seem long, much has happened since that time. Techniques have been improved, new types of equipment provided. A multidisciplinary approach has evolved, bringing together pathologists, diagnostic radiologists, radiation therapists, surgeons, internists, medical oncologists, obstetricians and gynecologists, geneticists, and others. Many radiologists and technologists have been trained in thermography, mammography, and xeroradiography; and a better understanding of the diagnosis and management of the patient with breast cancer has emerged.

The American College of Radiology breast program under the leadership of Wendell G. Scott, M.D. deserves great credit for having stimulated the development of xeroradiography, for encouraging training, and for emphasizing the importance of multidisciplinary cooperation in breast cancer control.

Today, every physician is bombarded with statistics that attempt to portray one method of therapy as superior to another. Continued publication of reports of experience will accomplish nothing unless *new* methods of diagnosis or treatment are presented. Best of all would be the determination of how to prevent breast cancer. The prognostic significance of the tumor type, of the stage of the disease, of the size of the cancer and its location, of its nuclear grade, of the degree of lymph node reactivity and of lymphoid infiltration in breast cancer must be considered. Careful attention must be directed to the other breast, since the same stimulus that caused the breast cancer affects all the mammary tissue.

A volunteer organization such as the American Cancer Society has great potential in the eventual control of cancer. This organization has the capacity to act quickly, independently, and with flexibility. For example, because breast cancer is the most prevalent cancer in women (90,000 new cases will be diagnosed in 1974 and there will be 33,000 deaths), in September 1971 it was decided that a program to combat this disease should be initiated by the Society. Within six months, the Society developed, implemented, and partially funded a major program to diagnose breast cancer at the earliest possible stage.

The earlier diagnosis of breast cancer can now be achieved by a combination of clinical examination, thermography, and mammography or xeroradiography. Public education programs and professional education programs are being expanded. Training programs for radiologists and technologists in the use of the newer techniques are being encouraged. More important, the American Cancer Society is cosponsoring with the National Cancer Institute 27 Breast Cancer Detection Projects, each to screen annually 5000 asymptomatic women over 35 years of age. Women participating will be taught breast self-examination. Many radiologists and technologists will receive training in thermography, mammography, or xeroradiography. This program is an excellent example of the potential of cooperative endeavor between a voluntary organization and the Federal government.

The American Cancer Society is delighted to be a cosponsor of this annual conference with the American College of Radiology and the National Cancer Institute. I know of no other conference on a continuing basis that has done so much for the control of breast cancer.

JUSTIN J. STEIN, M.D.

Preface

The papers in this volume were originally presented at the Thirteenth Annual Conference on Detection and Treatment of Early Breast Cancer in March 1974. Some were submitted as formal manuscripts, others were reconstructed from verbatim transcripts of the proceedings. Each presentation has been edited to reduce repetition and to emphasize the author's major points. By this procedure it has been possible to organize a large volume of diverse information into a compact, concise unit.

Much of the actual work involved in this process was done by my wife and favorite collaborator, Bette W. Gallager. It was she who reduced the hundreds of pages of the transcript to workable size and who patiently typed and retyped each chapter through its numerous revisions. She also assumed responsibility for the preparation of the manuscript for the publisher, corrected the proofs, and prepared the index. Her skill, her tireless effort, and her enthusiasm for the task have made my part of it easy.

Thanks are due to the Committee on Mammography and Diseases of the Breast of the American College of Radiology, who arranged the conference and to the American Cancer Society (Grant M.G. No. 176A) and the National Cancer Institute (Contract NC1-CN-55217), whose grants supported it financially. Particularly deserving of recognition is Robert W. Harrington, Ph.D., Director of Education of the American College of Radiology, without whose skillful management the conference would never have taken place, and without whose energetic support this book would never have been completed.

Houston, Texas   H. STEPHEN GALLAGER, M.D.
July 1975

Contents

Contents

EARLY BREAST CANCER

PART ONE

DEFINING THE PROBLEM

Mammography:
A Historical Perspective

ROBERT L. EGAN, M.D.

Mammography has done more to influence the diagnosis and treatment of breast cancer than any other event of the past six decades. It was introduced at a time when 95% of breast cancers were discovered by patients themselves; when women delayed seeking medical attention because of fear; when physicians were missing 25% of these relatively advanced cancers on initial examination. There was no satisfactory classification of breast diseases despite voluminous literature. There was great controversy as to definitive and even palliative treatment. Almost complete lack of knowledge of the natural history of this cancer prevailed. Rapport among patient, referring physician, surgeon, radiologist, and pathologist was minimal.

Mammography had barely passed through the stage of laboratory investigation into routine adjunctive diagnostic use before this began to change. Surgeons showed keen interest in prebiopsy mammographic histologic diagnoses, and soon developed enough confidence to explore mammographically suspicious areas in clinically normal breasts. Pathologists soon learned that problems in localization of breast lesions were reduced. Failure to find histopathologic confirmation of mammographic lesions led to more careful study of specimens and, inevitably, routine breast speciman radiography followed. This was at first applied to biopsy specimens, but soon there was added correlated x-ray and histologic study of mastectomy specimens.

These correlated studies have shown that no more than 1 in 20 breast

---

For details of the history of mammography see R. L. Egan, *Mammography*, 2nd ed., Springfield: Charles C. Thomas, 1972.

cancers corresponds to the fossilized concept of a mass with or without metastasis to the axillary lymph nodes. Cancer of the breast must be considered a whole organ disease. The carcinomas are usually multiple, often of different histologic types and readily metastasize within the breast. Intraductal noninvasive carcinoma is found in every breast containing invasive carcinoma, usually nearby as well as distant.

Breast cancer proceeds through an orderly, indolent progression of ductal hyperplasia, anaplasia, preinvasion, and invasion. This knowledge justifies the search for a method of identifying the point of irreversibility of this process.

According to Wendell G. Scott, "Mammography has done more to stimulate interest in breast cancer than any single procedure since the introduction of the radical mastectomy by Halsted." New ideas and procedures have been generated. The development of the team approach to the management of breast cancer is one significant breakthrough. As Dr. Lauren V. Ackerman observed at the Sixth Annual Symposium, "It is a tremendous accomplishment to get surgeons, radiologists, and pathologists in the same room, a greater one to get them to exchange ideas, and incredible that each would expose his limitations and invite his colleagues' help with breast cancer."

Mammography, not being absolute, has stimulated application of other procedures to breast diagnosis, among them ionography, radioisotope scanning, thermography, ultrasonography, and xeroradiography. It has revived interest in breast self-examination. It has led to these seminars, among which the Eighth Annual Symposium on Mammography and Diseases of the Breast was the largest conference on breast cancer ever held.

After a number of distinguished physicians visited M.D. Anderson Hospital following the 1960 Egan report on mammography, Dr. Lewis C. Robbins, Chief of the Cancer Control Program, Public Health Service, concluded: "The surgeons in this institution have learned to use mammography as a prebiopsy aid, and their confidence lends additional credence to the Egan report. The results are evidence of a real and tangible breakthrough. But one cannot accept this evidence if other radiologists cannot duplicate these results."

There followed an unprecedented nationwide reproducibility study, the first such study in the history of medicine. This study demonstrated that radiologists with five days of indoctrination could perform satisfactory mammography and led the Surgeon General of the United States to conclude, "Mammography shows promise of being an important diagnostic aid in the control of cancer of the breast."

As a result of mammography, much has improved. There has sprung up a more uniform terminology for breast diseases. Pathologists generally are less ready to throw specimens away, and even admit they are not 100% accurate. The radiologic technologists have been elevated to the stature of indispensable members of the team. Technical people and manufacturers now listen and heed advice. A new dimension has been added to radiology with low KVP, high MAS, and fine grain film techniques for other applications, such as rheumatology. In some areas 80% of operable breast cancers now have no axillary node involvement and 92% of nonpalpable cancers are node free. Of cancers evidenced only by calcifications in mammograms, 98 to 99% have no axillary node metastasis. There is an entirely new appeal to women exemplified by the ACS-NCI demonstration projects. Haagensen notes that in the last 15 years the average patient delay has dropped from seven and one half to five months. Women are seeking more complete evaluation prior to submitting to surgery. Many are actually demanding the right to mammography—among other rights. More breasts are being biopsied, but the ratio of malignant to benign remains the same. Fewer radical operative procedures are being done and cure rate of breast cancer is being increased. Today's improved mammograms allow the radiologist to go beyond simple diagnosis to the evaluation of unique shadows and more meaningful understanding of breast diseases.

Mammography is unquestionably our most productive means for screening populations for breast cancer. Some centers are reporting discovery rates of 8 to 14 cancers per 1000 women screened. No one can possibly predict the impact that screening will have. Relatively few women in the United States will be screened in the demonstration projects, but each can be expected to stir up interest in other women, thereby forcing more attention by the members of the medical profession.

The computer will have two tremendous roles in breast cancer detection. The first will be the placement of women into relative risk groups by evaluation of multiple indicators. Thermography will be important among the predictive factors. The second role of the computer will be in electronic evaluation of mammograms.

These hints of progress only serve as an indication of the real impact of mammography: it has revealed how little we know about breast cancer and how much there is to learn.

Mammography— An Assessment of Its Present Capabilities

THOMAS CARLILE, M.D.

The observations presented are based on some 12 years of experience in mammography and involvement in a screening center for the last six months. Between private practice and the screening center, we have reached a total experience in excess of 30,000 examinations. Thus any errors that I commit cannot be attributed to lack of opportunity to observe and learn.

Initially, it is easy to be complacent about how far we have come in mammography. The more one delves into the subject, however, the more concerned he becomes about how much we do not know. Mammography is emerging from childhood into adolescence with all of the attendant problems. A beginning has been made, but a mature system with most factors fully developed and under control is still in the future.

The present capabilities of mammography are limited by lack of ideal x-ray units and processing systems. We need units capable of operating in the upright position to allow high volume. They must produce images of the entire breast, including the back of the breast, as shown by inclusion of the rib cage, at an acceptable radiation dosage. At present the best imaging is done with multiple views in both upright and horizontal positions, allowing a workload of from 14 to 15 patients a day. This load could at least be doubled by a well-designed upright unit.

Present imaging systems are not optimal from the standpoint of detail and reliability. One must abandon industrial film and manual processing with its exceptional detail to increase capacity. The newer films that permit automatic processing and the vacuum pack single screen system represent efforts to overcome the above problems at some sacrifice of image quality. The selenium plate-paper image system has reliability problems as the processors are used for larger numbers of patients. Xeroradiographs can be read more rapidly, comfortably, and confidently when the correct technique has been achieved and when the processors are working well. Fortunately, the efforts of the manufacturers to improve reliability and service are rapidly producing results.

From the standpoint of our ability to interpret images, we seem to be approaching the visual limits in pattern and element recognition. Martin's review of January 1973 reported three carcinomas of 3 mm size; Scranton reports consistent recognition of particles in a phantom at 0.2 mm and Egan at 0.05 mm.

The ability to recognize these small masses, fibrils, and calcifications is inevitably wrapped up in image quality. Poor imaging and inability to recognize it can be responsible for not seeing significant lesions, leading to delay in diagnosis and also discrediting mammography and preventing it from fulfilling its present capabilities. As an example of this, when we first started using xeroradiography with a molybdenum tube, the images were so underpenetrated that the obvious solution seemed to be to increase kilovoltage. Finally we were using 48 to 55 kV with, of course, a corresponding reduction in milliampere seconds. This combination provided a far better image than the technique using 38 kV. In more recent work, however, it became apparent that the image at 50 kV and above suffered in detail when compared to a 38 kV image with appropriate milliampere seconds. The problem, then, was underexposure due to lack of milliampere seconds rather than underpenetration. However, it then became evident in dosimetry studies that the superior 38 kV image was achieved only at the expense of doubling the dose to the breast.

In the opinion of many, the tungsten anode tube produces a better xeroradiographic image than does the molybdenum anode tube, even with aluminum filtration rather than a molybdenum filter. This has not been tested under conditions of identical equipment and geometry. Thanks to the CGR Corporation, who provided us with a tungsten tube to work in a Senograph, and also to the Washington Division of the American Cancer Society, who provided us with a second Senograph, we can now do studies on the same patient with identical geometry in two units in the same room using a tungsten anode tube in one and a molybdenum anode tube in the other. In this way, we are able to compare image quality and radiation dose with different combinations of the two tubes and filters. All of this work is being done with xeroradiographic imaging, since previous experience has established the superiority of the molybdenum target with film.

This work is in progress and impressions are preliminary. Early results suggest that the 50 kV molybdenum anode-aluminum filter image is less satisfactory than either the 38 kV molybdenum anode-aluminum filter image or the tungsten anode-aluminum filter image. On blind testing of a relatively small number of images by three other radiologists, the impression is substantiated that in most cases the 38 kV molybdenum anode image is superior to the tungsten anode image. This is not always true, and in a significant number of cases the tungsten image is picked as the most desirable. The factor of the greatest importance probably will be dosage. The tungsten anode image, which is almost as good as and sometimes better than the corresponding molybdenum anode image, can be produced at half the radiation dose. Although this is a work-in-progress report, it seems unlikely that the total compilation of data will change these conclusions.

The xeroradiographic system has had great difficulty in providing sustained operation under the high volume conditions encountered in screening centers. As a result of discussions with members of the Committee on Mammography of the American College of Radiology and the project directors of the screening centers, the manufacturers have developed a program of providing backup units where needed and instituting a preventive maintenance program, which holds promise of providing increased reliability and constancy of imaging. In addition, recognizing the importance of quality of technique, a national program of technologists' seminars has been developed with aids to recognize an optimal image and how to achieve it.

Let us assume that by some good fortune we had reliable equipment producing excellent images consistently. Under the assumed circumstances, what is the present capability of mammography in relation to providing service by experienced radiologists operating at a high level of competence? Again, much is to be desired, but it is highly encouraging to see the progress that has been made in the past few years. There are a number of interwoven factors that have to advance together to produce the optimum effect: first, interest on the part of radiologists; second, acceptance by clinicians; third, adequate volume to permit development of expertise; fourth, accuracy at a level that develops confidence in the system; fifth, an interested pathologist and facilities for specimen radiography; and last, possibly that good stroke of fortune that convinces a skeptical surgeon early in his experience that nonpalpable, occult carcinoma does exist and can be diagnosed. I would prefer to leave the problem of the reluctant surgeon to others and talk about the radiologist.

The present capability of mammograpy is severely limited by the lack of radiologists who have had enough training or experience to be comfortable with the technique and promote its wider acceptance. Only in the last year has there been a definite move to include mammography in the examinations of the American Board of Radiology. Once this word gets around to

Thermographic Examination of the Breast: An Assessment of Its Present Capabilities

J. D. WALLACE

From the strict viewpoint of a physicist, it is axiomatic that infrared scanning, thermography, is incapable of detecting carcinoma of the breast. Infrared scanning techniques *are* capable of detecting variations in the absolute radiation flux in a given band as a function of location. Nowhere in this statement of capability is there any mention of human breasts or cancer. It matters not at all whether the radiation comes from a distant star or the tail of a comet, from a tank hidden in the jungle or a blast furnace, from the effluent of a power plant, from a printed computer circuit, or from the breasts of a female patient.

This, then, indicates that thermography as we usually know it—that is, scanning—provides a pictorial representation of the variations in the radiant flux taken in a given band from whatever surface is beng investigated. Note that the word *surface* is used. In the case of solids, radiation originates solely from the surface. In the early days of thermography the question constantly posed by clinicians was "How deep does it see?" The constant answer to that question was then, is now, and will forever be that thermography sees only the surface. In contradistinction to roentgenographic techniques, thermography simply maps the surface, and in that aspect is somewhat similar to human vision in that the human eye also sees only the surface.

When a physician looks at a patient he often sees surface manifestations due to underlying disease—pallor, cyanosis, or erythema, for instance. That

13

the surface temperature of the human body or any reasonable segment of it is not uniform is a reasonable assumption, and this, of course, has been the regular finding in thermography by which such variations are easily visualized. In his first report, Lawson, who originated medical thermography, indicated that he based his investigations on the premise that in malignant processes there was "accelerated local metabolism" that could be detected by estimating the change in temperature caused by the tumor in its immediate environment. It would not be unreasonable to expect that inflammatory and other benign processes characterized by high metabolic rates could produce similar changes in temperature in their immediate environments.

All of this brings us back to the physicist's point of view: it is axiomatic that thermography is incapable of diagnosing carcinoma of the breast. Infrared techniques are able and are expressly designed to detect variations in the absolute radiation flux in a given band as a function of location. The foregoing, of course, are the strict statements of a physicist. Having established this foundation, let us go on to more practical problems. That the variations in radiation flux as a function of location on the human body are influenced by conditions under the skin is also axiomatic. It therefore behooves us to look into, among other things, the mechanism by which this influence is exercised.

Cooper, Randall, and Hertzman some years ago described their physiologic studies of the transport of excess heat from active muscle to the overlying skin. The effects of exercise of the arms was studied during rhythmic manual compression of a rubber bulb. They observed the skin temperature of the forearm during periods of exercise and at rest. Based on these experiments, it was concluded that (a) "A significant fraction of the heat generated in rhythmically contracting muscle may be transferred by vascular convection along vertical channels, which either traverse the muscle or connect its vascular system with that of the overlying skin," and that (b) "The direct nonconvective transfer of the extra heat appearing in the overlying skin is relatively less important." Cooper and his associates found that there was no increase in skin temperature over exercising muscles while compression was applied. When the compression was released, the temperature of the skin over the muscle rose rapidly and immediately. This was considered evidence that the principal mode of the transfer of heat from deep structures to the skin is that of venous convection.

In a recent article Dodd and his co-workers suggested that the mechanism of heat transfer may, in fact, be dependent on the depth of the source of the abnormal heat. Conduction may predominate for sources that are superficially located and involve the skin, whereas venous convection is the principal mode for deeply seated sources. Whether all excess heat is carried to the surface in the manner suggested by Cooper, or whether, more logically, it is a function of location, nowhere in these studies is any exclusivity assigned in the mechanism to malignant processes.

In addition to "accelerated local metabolism," thermal patterns may be produced on the skin by environmental influences and by humanly produced artifacts.

Figure 1 is a thermogram of an asymptomatic woman. Note that, in the main, the right breast is warmer than the left. Or is it that the left breast is cooler than the right? In fact, this woman was thermographed with an air conditioning draft playing directly on her left breast. This is an example of environmental influence that, in this instance, produced a cooling artifact. If the air had been warm or if she had been in the radiant field of a hot radiator, there would have been a hot artifact.

Figure 2 illustrates, in the upper inner quadrant of the right breast, an unusual radiating venous pattern. Such a pattern should heighten suspicion. This lady was particularly modest and placed her hand over the upper inner

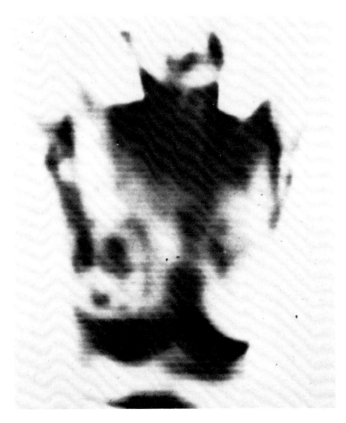

Figure 1

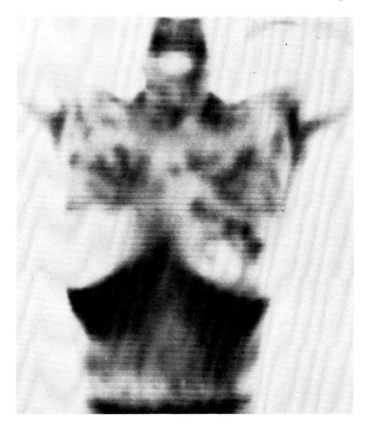

Figure 2

quadrant of her right breast during cooling. This, then, is an example of a
humanly produced artifact.

Figure 3 shows two thermograms made one year apart. The development
of a highly abnormal venous pattern in the later examination is clearly
apparent and highly suspicious. This abnormal pattern is due to a condition
that often strikes females in their twenties—pregnancy.

Figure 4 is the thermogram of a female with a mass in the right breast. The
thermographic pattern is highly abnormal. There is an abnormal venous
pattern that radiates from an abnormally hot areola. This lady had a large
fibroadenoma.

Scanners have been improved both in picture quality and price. To date,
however, there is no study that suggests that either high picture quality or
lower cost have brought about significant improvement in clinical performance as far as breast cancer screening is concerned.

Ghys has reviewed the literature and assembled the reported experience
in 38,500 cases (Table 1). In this group there were 2236 histologically

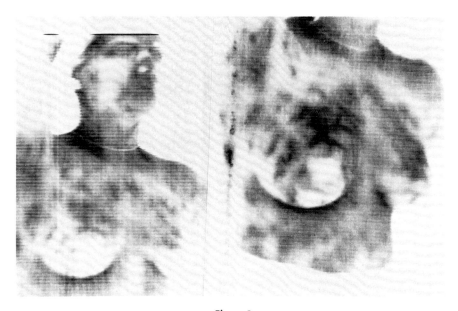

Figure 3

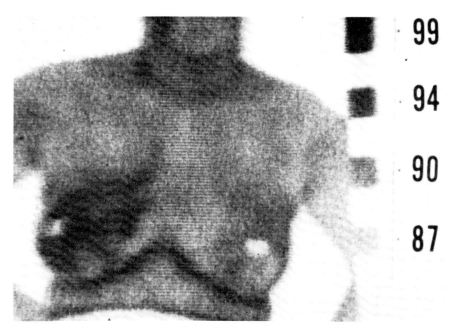

Figure 4

Table 1: Accumulated Experience with Thermography (Ghys)

Year of Publication	Principal Author	Number of Cases	Cancers Verified Historically	Thermography +	Thermography −	Positives (%)	False Negatives (%)
1965	SWEARINGEN	100	19	19	0	100	0
1965	BRASFIELD	150	38	25	13	66	34
1966	HARRIS	100	60	53	7	89	11
1966?	SEAMAN	?	80	63	17	79	21
1967	GERSHON-COHEN	4 000	200	188	12	94	6
1967	HOFFMAN	1 924	24	18	6	75	25
1968	HITCHCOCK	2 523	4	1	3	25	75
1968	BUCHWALD	200	34	24	10	70.5	29.5
1968	MELANDER	> 1 400	281	262	19	93.2	6.8
1969	ISARD	2 696	76	55	21	72	28
1969?	MADSEN	173	8	6	2	75	25
1969	WALLACE	4 726	195	166	29	85	15
1969	SAMUEL	193	78	48	30	61.5	38.5
1969	WILLIAMS	300	167	153	14	91.6	8.4
1969	SHAWE	738	3	3	0	100	0
1969	HESSLER	400	34	28	6	82.4	17.6
1969	LILIENFELD (6 diagnostic centers)	3 511	305	226	79	74.1	25.9
1970	GHYS	275	2	2	0	100	0
1970	GROS [b]	6 000	272 [a]	247	25	90.5	9.5
1971	AARTS [b]	236	93	90	3	97	3
1972	AMALRIC	1 500	226	209	17	93	7
1972	MELANDER	7 200	37 [c]	33	4	89	11
Total		> 38 500	2 236	1 919	317	86	14

[a] In 10 bilateral cases.
[b] Personal communication.
[c] Eleven precancerous conditions and 58 benign tumors were also uncovered and biopsied.

confirmed cancers of the breast and the thermograms were suspicious in 1919 instances, yielding a true positive rate of 86%.

In a recent article Dodd et al. stated that "thermographic examination can be expected to detect at least three of four breast malignancies" and that "screening procedures using an unselected group of asymptomatic patients, age 35 years or more, will usually result in an overall false positive rate of 12 to 15%."

Thus we have two important inputs from which to project the expected performance of thermography in screening for female breast cancer: (a) the technique can be expected to be suspicious in 75 to 86% of patients with carcinoma of the breast, and (b) in screening asymptomatic women 12 to 15% of the thermographic examinations will be suspicious.

If we assume, as Strax et al. have reported, that in mammographic screening the incidence of breast cancer is 2.72 per 1000, then the expected cancer rate among thermographically suspicious patents can be calculated. Combining the Ghys performance figure with the Strax incidence and a false positive rate of 12 to 15%, the expected rate among patients with suspicious thermograms would range from 19.5 to 15.6 per 1000. If we assume the less optimistic performance figure of 75%, the rates become 17 to 13.6 per 1000 suspicious thermograms, respectively.

It has been predicted that there will be about 89,000 new cases of breast cancer in the United States this year. These cancers will occur within an at-risk population of about 33 million women. By screening these women thermographically, it would seem possible to select from the 33 million 4 to 5 million women in whom would be found between 66,000 and 76,000 of the cancers.

It is pertinent at this juncture to recall that thermography is a relatively inexpensve procedure performed by a technician. It imposes no radiation burden on the patient and requires no physical contact with the patient. The resulting thermogram contains only a small amount of information as compared with a mammogram, so that the reading of thermograms is a substantially simpler task.

It seems to me that the role of thermography in breast cancer detection is that of initial screening. Beyond that, its lack of specificity at this stage in its development makes more extensive use unwarranted. If a simple, innocuous technique can concentrate the sought population by a significant factor, and if this is deemed a useful contribution, then thermography has a role and the population it selects can then be further examined using the more specific methods.

Changes in Surgical Practice as a Result of Mammography and Thermography

ASHBEL C. WILLIAMS, M.D.
MARVIN V. McCLOW, M.D.

To those who have more than a passing interest in breast cancer and considerably more than the average physician's knowledge of it, mammography, xeroradiography, and thermography have become household terms and accepted procedures, the advantages of which are obvious. In many communities, however, such an attitude is not prevalent, but is limited to those indiviuals and groups who have informed themselves in the technical and clinical aspects of this relatively new field of medical expertise. Attitudes are changing, however, because of the intensification of the educational activities of the American College of Radiology, the American Cancer Society, and the Cancer Control Program of the Federal Government.

It has been of great interest to observe in our own medical community the process of orientation of the medical profession toward mammography. Soon after the emergence of modern mammography, it became obvious that the radiologist, the surgeon, and the pathologist should work together as a team, consulting relative to the details of each patient's problem. Perhaps radiologists have most often been responsible for kindling interest in mammography locally, but surgeons have also ignited the spark in many situations. The experiences to be related are perhaps unique in that they show the development of a mammography program in a community hospital with no direct connection with a medical school or a large research institution.

At the outset, surgeons in our community were skeptical. Confidence in mammography came slowly. Conversion usually was consummated only as each surgeon experienced having a patient's unsuspected carcinoma revealed by a mammogram. Over the 11 years since the initiation of mammography of St. Vincent's Medical Center, the physician interest and participation have risen gratifyingly. In December 1972 we reported our first 10 years' experience, a study of 4030 mammographic examinations. In the 15 months since then, 2566 additional mammograms have been performed, more than half the number done in the first 10 years!

In early December 1973 the St. Vincent's Breast Diagnostic Center was opened as 1 of the 27 centers established during the past year and supported by the National Cancer Institute and the American Cancer Society. In order to meet the required quota of 5000 examinations per year, over 20 patients are being screened each work day. In addition, 10 to 15 mammographic examinations per day are performed on referred symptomatic women. Conventional mammography has given way to xeromammography. Each examinee also has a thermogram.

To assess the impact that mammography has exerted on surgical practice, we focus on several new developments and trends we have observed.

Most striking is the dramatic increase in the number of breast biopsies, 149 having been performed in 1969 as compared with 309 in 1973, an increase of 109%! There has also been a marked increase in mammary resections of various types for primary breast cancer, 52 such operations having been performed in 1969 and 83 in 1973, an increase of 63%. Since the total number of surgical operations performed at St. Vincent's Medical Center increased only 20% between 1969 and 1973, it is apparent that this upsurge in biopsies and breast resections reflects a new awakening to the problem, more careful attention to breast lesions, and a broadening of the indications for biopsy. Fundamental to this escalation in activity is the motivating influence exerted by mammography on the surgeon as well as on the patient.

At St. Vincent's 45 patients underwent mastectomies with nodal dissections in 1969. Axillary nodes were negative in 27 patients (60%) and positive in 18 (40%). In 1973 there were 73 mastectomies with nodal dissections and the percentage of nodal involvement was exactly the same as in 1969. There was one significant difference, however. Among the patients with negative nodes in 1969 there were two who had noninfiltrating cancers. In 1973 there were 9 patients with in situ cancer. Since all of these cases were discovered through mammography, this shift toward diagnosis of the disease in a curable stage should appropriately be credited to mammography. We are of the opinion that, as the patients undergoing mammography in our Breast

Diagnostic Center shift from predominantly symptomatic to predominantly asymptomatic, we will encounter fewer positive mammograms, but the lesions discovered will show a definite trend toward greater curability.

In our previous study among 3030 mammographic examinations over a 10 year period, 191 cancers were discovered, a yield of 6.2%. In the 15 months since that report, 2566 mammographic examinations have been done and 76 cancers have been discovered, a yield of 3.6%. The preponderance of the cancers in both groups was found by mammography, those missed being suspected on palpation.

During the 15 month period ended January 31, 1974 there were 76 patients who had mammograms prior to surgery and who were found to have primary breast cancer. Of these 76 patints, 61 or 80% were diagnosed or suspected by mammography. In 15 patients (20%) the diagnosis was missed on mammography. The percentage of diagnoses missed on mammography in an earlier series was 11%. On physical examination, 60 of the 76 patients (79%) were diagnosed or suspected clinically. In 16 cases (21%) the tumor was missed on clinical examination but diagnosed by mammography, a figure almost identical to that in our previous report. These tumors we refer to as occult, since they were not clinically manifest and would have been overlooked except for mammography. In our previous study 18.3% of the tumors were occult. It is necessary then, to have both meticulous physical examination and mammography to reach maximal diagnostic efficiency.

Of the patients who had mammography followed by surgery, positive nodes were found in 35%. This compares with a rate of 40% in all patients operated on for primary breast cancer during the same period. Mammography may have led to operation at a more favorable stage.

Of the patients whose tumors were missed on physical examination, five, or 31%, had positive nodes. In those cases in which the lesions were missed by mammography, there were positive nodes in five instances (37%). These sobering figures suggest that our best efforts are none too good. The ultimate policy should be to screen women in the appropriate age group when they are both sign and symptom free to detect truly early lesions. For individuals in high risk categories our best efforts should be intensified.

There were 24 biopsies performed on the basis of suspicious mammographic findings and reported as benign. This constitutes a "false positive" rate of 0.9%.

In our community, the great bulk of mammographic examinations are performed at St. Vincent's Medical Center, thus encouraging the development in that hospital of a degree of technical and professional expertise that comes only from experience and is essential to acceptable accuracy.

In the surgical practice of one of us, mammographic records have been kept since May 1968. From that date to February 1974, a period of five and one-half years, 726 patients were referred for mammograms. Occult cancers were detected in 9 of these patients, or 1.2%. At surgery, positive lymph nodes were present in only 1 patient.

Several additional developments relating to our breast program deserve mention. About 18 months ago, a self-contained radiographic unit was acquired so that biopsy specimens can be subjected to immediate radiography in the operating suite. Then, in cases where the lesion is not palpable, it can be determined whether the area under suspicion has been included in the biopsy or whether additional tissue must be removed. Specimen radiography in such cases is essential to guide the pathologist to assure that he sections the lesion. Also, an occasional unsuspected lesion may be discovered by this technique. Quadrant sized biopsy specimens are usually taken when the lesion is occult. It is mandatory that the radiologist localize the lesion as accurately as possible preoperatively and equally mandatory that the surgeon consult personally with the radiologist so that both are fully oriented before surgery.

In a few cases, when the clinical examination has been strongly suggestive of carcinoma and the mammogram equally positive, clinical considerations have led to mastectomy without biopsy. In such instances, the surgeon must be prepared to justify his action with convincing clinical data. While this procedure is occasionally permissible, it is our firm policy that mammography not be used as a substitute for biopsy and that mammographic evidence be histologically substantiated before radical surgery is performed.

After reviewing the records of several hundred operations for primary breast cancer in our community hospital, the impression is gained that there is a recent tendency toward simple mastectomies and so-called modified radical mastectomies. Some surgeons are tending to perform less-than-radical mastectomy if a breast lesion is small or otherwise favorable. In a number of studies, it has been pointed out that nodal metastases can and do occur when the primary is disarmingly small. Several patients in this review developed nodal disease after limited surgery and axillary dissection was necessitated at a later date. Patients with minimal disease should have full resections, as they are the most highly curable if given the benefit of adequate resection and thorough nodal dissection. Complete removal of axillary nodes by "modified radical mastectomy" is technically more difficult than by standard radical mastectomy. In the hands of those with extensive knowledge and technical expertise, there is a definite place for the modified radical mastectomy, so long as the procedure does not compromise the completeness of the nodal resection. The term "modified radical mastectomy," however, has many meanings, and for the occasional mastectomist it may well serve as a cover for an inadequate resection.

Thermographic findings have not been discussed because, in the experience of our department of radiology, this modality has not yet produced sufficient accuracy and consistency to be dependable. For statistical and technical experience, thermography is performed on every patient having a mammogram.

In summary, our breast cancer diagnostic program is very much on the upswing with constantly increasing tempo, volume, and interest. The final evaluation of this increased activity must await the careful analysis of additional 10 year follow-ups in substantial numbers before we can ascertain if and how much survival rates have been improved. The statistics now beginning to come in indicate that we are on the right track.

Meanwhile we have good reason to urge the wider use of mammography, the complete removal of the breast and regional lymph nodes when cancer is diagnosed, and the keeping of meticulous records so that an accurate conclusion may be reached when this material comes of age.

Estrogens, the Pill, and the Breast

LAMAN A. GRAY, M.D.
ROBERT W. ROBERTSON, Jr., M.S.

No complete explanation of the effect of ovarian hormones on the human breast exists, but the general opinion persists that estrogens stimulate ductal epithelium and periductal connective tissue, and that progesterone probably stimulates acinar epithelium. Progestins, as in contraceptive hormonal combinations, also affect ductal epithelium and may produce sclerosis of intralobular connective tissues. Prolactin from the pituitary gland is also a stimulating factor.

Estrogens have been implicated as a possible cause of breast cancer in animals since the original work of Loeb in 1919. Only sporadic reports of estrogen related breast cancer in humans have appeared up to the present. Hertz in 1967 reported that there were only four prior studies, including 120 to 292 women each, of patients receiving estrogens. There was no apparent increase in breast cancer in these groups. Hertz warned that this was limited data and that long term studies were necessary. In 1970 Gray reported that of 1085 women who received oral estrogens, 20 developed breast cancer after an average period of estrogenic therapy of nine years. Burch and Byrd reported a series of 511 women followed nine or more years, among whom 9 developed carcinoma of the breast. This incidence was considered to be the same as that to be anticipated among women of comparable age without hormone therapy.

That nodular thickenings and painful areas in the breast are related to ovarian hormones is demonstrated by the variation of such symptoms with the menstrual cycle and by their disappearance after menopause. Evidently both estrogens and progesterone are implicated. After the menopause and after all thickening has disappeared, estrogens may be given in small dosages to patients with prior breast complaints without stimulation of the breasts, except in a small percentage (4.9%). Macrocysts occur predominantly in the premenopausal period and ordinarily do not recur after menopause when estrogens are essentially absent. With estrogenic therapy for menopausal symptoms, macrocysts appear in 1.8%. A concern that estrogens may have some relationship to the development of breast cancer persists, and further statistical studies over long periods are needed.

The possibility that contraceptive hormonal preparations may cause breast cancer, perhaps many years later, has been mentioned by Hertz. Nodularities, engorgement, and mastalgia occur in patients taking birth control pills, but are only rarely severe. When such changes are marked, the medication should be discontinued.

Goldenberg, Wiegenstein, and Mottet described four cases of florid fibroadenomas in patients receiving birth control pills. Gray reported two similar tumors in patients who had been taking birth control pills and another in a woman who had never received any exogenous hormone. Fechner compared fibroadenomas from patients taking birth control preparations and those receiving no hormones and found no histologic differences. Similarly, Taylor found no special characteristics in fibrocystic disease of the breast in patients taking birth control pills as compared with those who had received no hormonal therapy. Fechner found that the tumors in five breast carcinoma patients taking birth control pills were not histologically distinctive.

In an effort to study further the effect of various steroids on breast lesions, the microscopic findings in a series of breast biopsies have been correlated with the information available as to hormone therapy. Microscopic slides from 850 consecutive breast biopsies done between November 1969 and July 1973 were reexamined. All of these biopsies were performed in the Norton-Children's Hospitals and represented areas of thickening or nodularity of concern to the patients and their physicians. Of the 850 patients, 320 (37.6%) had received no hormone therapy of any type. In 365 records (42.9%), there was no information as to whether the patients had received hormone therapy. Of the remaining 165 women (19.4%), 94 (11.0%) had been receiving estrogens and 71 (8.4%) oral contraceptive hormonal preparations (Table 1).

The histologic diagnoses of the 850 specimens included duct hyperplasia in 263 and sclerosing adenosis in 227. Florid adenosis was present in 12 biopsies and florid adenomas in 3. Fibroadenomas were found in 166, benign cysts in 167, while various degrees of inflammation about the ducts and acini occurred in 125. Interlobular sclerosis was present in 272 patients

Table 1   Hormonal Treatment Status in 850 Consecutive Patients Undergoing Breast Biopsy, NOVEMBER 1969—JULY 1973

No hormone therapy		320
Hormone therapy		165
Estrogens	94	
Birth control pills	71	
No information		365

and fat and atrophy in 303. Carcinoma was found in 178 (20.9%). More than one diagnosis was included in many of these individual biopsies (Table 2).

Of the 178 patients with breast carcinomas, Paget's disease of the nipple occurred in 6 and carcinoma of mammary duct origin in 164. The latter were subdivided into 5 noninfiltrating and 159 infiltrating (Table 3). Carcinoma of lobules was present in 8 specimens, noninfiltrating in 3, and infiltrating in 5. Associated hyperplastic changes included duct hyperplasia in 53, sclerosing adenosis in 39, florid adenosis in 3, and intraductal papillomas in 16. Atrophic changes included interlobular sclerosis in 54 and fat and atrophy in 53 cases.

Estrogenic therapy was known to have been given to 94 of the 850 patients, generally for long periods. The average age of the treated patients was 56 years. Microscopic findings in their biopsies included carcinomas in 25 (Table 4). Benign lesions were found in the remainder. These included duct hyperplasia in 40, sclerosing adenosis in 12, florid adenosis in 2, and florid adenoma in 1. Intraductal papillomas were present in 12, intracystic

Table 2   Histologic Diagnoses in 850 Breast Biopsies

Duct hyperplasia	263 (30.9%)
Sclerosing adenosis	227 (26.7%)
Florid adenosis	12 (1.4%)
Florid adenoma	3 (0.4%)
Intraduct papilloma	61 (7.2%)
Intracystic papilloma	2 (0.3%)
Apocrine hyperplasia	41 (4.8%)
Adenoma of pregnancy	6 (0.7%)
Fibroadenoma	166 (19.5%)
Cyst	167 (19.6%)
Inflammation	125 (14.7%)
Carcinoma (all types)	178 (20.9%)
Interlobular sclerosis	272 (32.0%)
Fat and atrophy	303 (35.6%)

Table 3   Histologic Types of Breast Carcinomas Found in 850 Biopsies

Paget's disease of the nipple			6
Carcinoma of mammary ducts			164
Noninfiltrating		5	
Papillary	3		
Comedo	2		
Infiltrating		159	
Papillary	0		
Comedo	6		
Scirrhous	139		
Medullary	11		
Colloid	3		
Carcinoma of lobules			8
Noninfiltrating		3	
Infiltrating		5	
Total			178

Table 4   Histologic Diagnoses in 94 Breast Biopsies from Patients Receiving Estrogens

Duct hyperplasia		40 (42%)
Sclerosing adenosis		12 (13%)
Florid adenosis		2 (2%)
Intraduct papilloma		12 (13%)
Intracystic papilloma		2 (2%)
Apocrine hyperplasia		2 (2%)
Fibroadenoma		4 (4%)
Cyst		21 (22%)
Inflammation		19 (20%)
Carcinoma (all types)		25 (27%)
Duct	22	
Medullary	1	
Intraductal papillary	1	
Interlobular sclerosis		36 (38%)
Fat and atrophy		37 (39%)

papillomas in 1, fibroadenomas in 4, and benign cysts in 21. Atrophic changes, interlobular sclerosis and fat and atrophy, were present in 36 and 37 cases, respectively. The number of patients with hyperplastic lesions was almost equal to that of women with atrophic changes. There was no evidence that estrogens had uniformly stimulated the epithelium, although all of these patients had formed palpable breast lumps or thickenings.

Contraceptive hormonal preparations had been received by 71 of the patients, whose average age was 32 years (Table 5). Among these, 8 had carcinomas. Fibroadenomas were common, appearing in 27 of these younger patients (Figure 1). Duct hyperplasia was present in 24, sclerosing

Table 5 Histologic Diagnoses in 71 Breast Biopsies from Patients Receiving Contraceptive Pills

Duct hyperplasia		24 (34%)
Sclerosing adenosis		26 (37%)
Florid adenosis		2 (3%)
Intraduct papilloma		3 (4%)
Apocrine hyperplasia		5 (7%)
Fibroadenoma		27 (38%)
Cyst		6 (8%)
Inflammation		10 (14%)
Carcinoma		8 (11%)
Duct	6	
Comedo	1	
Medullary	1	
Interlobular sclerosis		25 (35%)
Fat and atrophy		6 (8%)

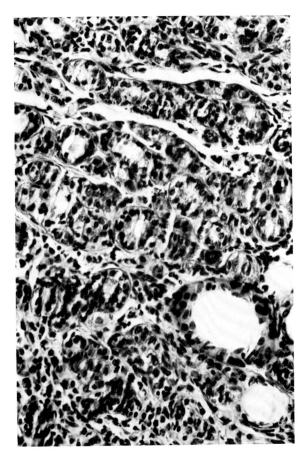

Figure 1 Breast biopsy from a 25 year old woman who was receiving contraceptive hormones. The lesion is an encapsulated fibroadenoma with florid adenosis.

adenosis in 26, florid adenosis in 2 (Figure 2), and intraductal papillomas in 3 patients. Interlobular sclerosis and fat and atrophy were present in 25 and 6 specimens, respectively. The hyperplastic changes in this group were somewhat more common than atrophic epithelial changes. The 8 carcinomas found in patients receiving contraceptive hormones represents the largest number yet reported.

Among the 320 patients known never to have received any hormonal preparations (37.6% of the total, with an average age of 45 years), carcinoma was present in 61. Duct hyperplasia was found in 97, sclerosing adenosis in 88, florid adenosis in 2 (Figure 3), and florid adenoma in 1. Intraductal papillomas were present in 17, intracystic papillomas in 1, and fibroadenomas in 58 patients. Other microscopic findings included atrophic changes of interlobular sclerosis in 98 and fat and atrophy in 95. The

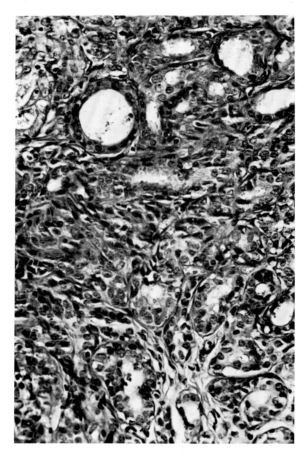

Figure 2   Breast biopsy from a woman, age 28, receiving contraceptive hormones. The sections show florid adenosis with cysts, papillomatosis, lobular hyperplasia, and a nonencapsulated fib roadenoma.

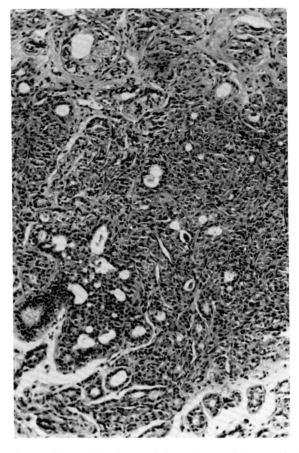

Figure 3   Biopsy from an 18 year old patient receiving no hormonal therapy. Florid adenosis and a noencapsulated fibroadenoma are present.

hyperplastic lesions slightly exceeded the atrophic changes in this group (Table 6).

When one compares patients known not to be receiving hormones with those taking birth control pills, the incidence of hyperplasia is similar (30.3% and 33.9%). On the other hand, of those receiving estrogens, 42.9% had duct hyperplasias. Carcinomas were found in 19% of those receiving no hormones, 26.6% of those receiving estrogens, and 11.2% of those taking birth control pills. The group taking birth control pills represented by far the youngest age group. Finally, of those with cancer and hyperplastic lesions, 36% had received no hormone, 28% had received estrogens, and 37.5% had taken birth control pills. This study indicates that there is no relationships to cancer. Of the patients biopsied who were receiving es-the hormonal status (Table 7).

A review of 850 breast biopsies has demonstrated that hyperplastic

Table 6   Histologic Diagnoses in 320 Breast Biopsies from Patients Receiving No Hormones

Duct hyperplasia	97 (30.3%)
Sclerosing adenosis	88 (27.5%)
Florid adenosis	2 (0.6%)
Florid adenoma	1 (0.3%)
Intraduct papilloma	17 (5.3%)
Intracystic papilloma	1 (0.3%)
Apocrine hyperplasia	14 (4.4%)
Adenoma of pregnancy	3 (0.9%)
Fibroadenoma	58 (18.1%)
Cyst	58 (18.1%)
Inflammation	41 (12.8%)
Carcinoma (all types)	61 (19.1%)
Interlobular sclerosis	98 (30.6%)
Fat and atrophy	95 (29.7%)

changes and atrophic changes occur with almost equal frequency in patients who received estrogenic hormone and those who did not. A like proportion appeared among patients who had breast cancer. Estrogenic hormonal therapy produced no characteristic microscopic changes suggestive of a relationship to cancer. Of the patients biopsied who were receiving estrogenic hormone, a larger percentage was found to have carcinoma, but the older median age of this group would seem to represent the significant factor.

No specific changes were found in the breasts of patients taking birth control hormonal preprations. Hyperplasias and sclerosing adenosis were not increased among those with malignancy. The lower percentage of cancer among patients in the birth control pill group is probably related to the younger age of these women. The long term effects of contraceptive hormonal therapy on the breast cannot be forecast at this time.

Our studies have led us to the following conclusions:

1. Among 850 breast biopsies histologically reviewed, hyperplastic and atrophic changes occurred with almost equal frequency. Rates were similar in patients who had received estrogenic hormone, those with no history of hormone therapy, and those who had breast cancer.
2. Estrogenic hormonal therapy produced no histologic changes suggesting a relationship to cancer. Of the 94 patients who were receiving estrogens, a larger percentage developed carcinoma, but the older median age of this group may explain this difference.
3. No specific changes were found in the breasts of 71 patients taking birth control hormonal preparations.

Table 7   Duct Hyperplasia and Carcinoma in 485 Breast Biopsies from Patients of Known Hormonal Status

Average Age	Number of Patients	Hormonal Therapy	Duct Hyperplasia	Carcinoma	Carcinoma with Hyperplasia
45	320	None	97 (30.3%)	61 (19%)	22 (36%)
56	94	Estrogen	40 (42.5%)	25 (26.6%)	7 (28%)
32	71	Oral contraceptives	24 (33.9%)	8 (11.2%)	3 (37.5%)

4. The younger women in the group had more hyperplastic changes than the older women. Twenty percent of all the biopsies showed cancer, but 42% of those from women over 55 contained cancer.

5. Estrogens are not a specific cause of hyperplasias in the breast. Neither they nor contraceptive hormonal preparations can at this time be considered to be major causes of breast cancer.

Women's Attitudes Regarding Breast Cancer: Results of the Gallup Poll

ARTHUR I. HOLLEB, M.D.

Several months ago the Gallup Organization, Inc. conducted a poll for the American Cancer Society. The study was designed to provide information that would be helpful in developing future plans and programs to increase public knowledge of an involvement with breast cancer and the newer methods for its detection and treatment.

The study was an in depth investigation of a variety of factors that might influence women's acceptance or rejection of early detection programs. Among the subject areas explored were breast self-examination, breast examination by physicians, women's attitudes toward the surgical treatment of breast cancer, factors that influence the acceptance by women of the current practice of mastectomy, and the signing of prior consent.

The specific objectives of the study were to seek answers to the following questions related to the early detection and surgical treatment of breast cancer:

1. What are the current medical care habits of women and how do they relate to the frequency with which women have their breasts examined?
2. How concerned are women about breast cancer and how well-informed are they regarding its prevalence, causes, and signs of its possible presence?
3. In what ways do embarrassment and the sex of physicians affect acceptance of breast examinations?

4. How aware are women of breast self-examination? How do they become aware of it and to what extent is awareness translated into actual practice?

5. How informed are women about how to do breast self-examination and how often it should be done? How does this compare with actual practice?

6. How confident are women that breast self-examination is an effective method for early detection of breast cancer?

7. What attitudes do women have about lumpectomy, simple mastectomy, and radical mastectomy; the need for extensive surgery; and the practice of obtaining prior consent?

8. What is the emotional impact of breast removal? How does this relate to marriage and one's sense of being a woman? What are the adjustment problems?

The study was designed as an in depth national survey of women 18 years of age and older. A national sample of 1007 women were individually questioned during interviews averaging one hour. A questionnaire was developed following a series of group discussions conducted qualitatively for refining the specific objectives of the study and for developing specific questions to ask in the survey. The demographic composition of each group was controlled to get representation of both younger and older women and women of high and low socioeconomic status.

To provide a detailed understanding of women's attitudes, beliefs, and practices, all survey results were analyzed by a variety of demographic and socioeconomic characteristics, as well as by a number of factors related to women's medical care habits. In addition, selected questions were analyzed in terms of a number of attitudinal and personality characteristics.

The final report is a document of nearly 150 pages of detailed analyses-—and it is an eye-opener for the medical profession and for those interested in public education. Here are just a few of the highlights that show how inadequate our educational efforts may have been and where our successes have been achieved.

Most women in the United States do not have their breasts examined by a physician with any frequency or regularity.

Cancer is the most salient health concern of women, and breast cancer figures prominently in this concern. No other health problem was named first by comparable percentages. Surprisingly, concern regarding breast cancer declines with age, and the greatest worry is found in women 18 to 34 years of age, those least likely to get breast cancer.

Women have an exaggerated idea of the prevalence of breast cancer. Only 8% gave a reasonably accurate estimate. This inflated notion was found in all segments of the population, including college educated and upper income groups.

Only 12% of all women know that most breast lumps are not cancer.

Optimism prevails about breast cancer treatment and only 5% believe that "very few" women survive. Older women are the most pessimistic.

Seventy-seven percent of all women know at least one woman who has had breast cancer.

Almost two-thirds of women believe that a blow or injury to the breast can produce breast cncer and less one-half know that a family history of breast cancer increases the chances that a woman might develop cancer herself.

About one-half of all women believe that birth control pills increase the chance of developing breast cancer.

Most women express no preference between seeing a male or female physician and 70% believe that male physicians really understand a woman's feeling about breast removal.

Embarrassment during breast examination can be reduced if the physician explains what he is doing and teaches breast self-examination.

Only one out of every four women who have heard of breast self-examination has ever practiced it, and three of four of these aware women do not practice it monthly.

Only 35% of all women report that a physician has ever *mentioned* the topic of breast self-examination to them, yet those who practice the technique are the ones who have been personally taught by physicians(92%).

There is no evidence at all that physicians stress the importance of monthly breast self-examination.

Virtually all women (96%) say that if breast cancer is detected early, the chances of cure are better. This is most encouraging.

When women were asked what they would do if they had a possible sign of cancer, 83% said they would go to a doctor immediately and 16% said they would wait to see if it would go away. Younger women showed a greater tendency to wait before seeing a physician.

Simple mastectomy was named by 34% as being the most frequently used breast cancer treatment and by 5% as the least. Radical mastectomy was named as used most often by 23% and least often by 36%. As for lumpectomy, 25% think it is used most often and 30% least often. This demonstrates the remarkable lack of knowledge American women have about current surgical management of breast cancer.

Simple mastectomy tends to be thought of as "extensive" surgery, whereas radical mastectomy is perceived as an "extreme" form of treatment.

As of now, women are far more confident about nonrecurrence of cancer if the entire breast is removed rather than only the lump. If only the cancerous lump were removed, 42% would be optimistic about nonrecurrence. In contrast, after breast removal 71% would be optimistic.

Women are almost equally divided in their opinions regarding prior consent for mastectomy: 48% are infavor of it and 45% want postdiagnostic discussion. Fear of returning to the operating room for a second operation, however, tends to dissipate the prior consent question. For younger women and unmarried women, the issue is not so much whether prior consent should be obtained but whether the breast must be removed.

Support for prior consent is strengthened if women have regular contact with physicians who perform breast examinations and if physicians discuss in detail, before exploratory surgery, what alternative therapeutic techniques exist and under what conditions a mastectomy would be performed.

Breast removal causes the expected emotional trauma but fear of a diagnosis of cancer contributes more to this trauma than does mastectomy itself.

Ninety-two percent of women think that a normal life pattern can be maintained or reestablished after a mastectomy, but there is less confidence among single and young women and among those of lower socioeconomic status.

These are but a few dominant features of the Gallup poll, but they are enough to show that we as physicians and health educators still have much to do. Breast cancer is the leading cancer killer of women in the United States and will probably remain so until two essential goals are reached: a better informed public and a medical profession alert to the need for personal instruction in breast self-examination, alert to the need for performing breast examinations whenever possible, and alert to the utilization of the newer modalities for the diagnosis of minimal breast cancer before a mass has appeared.

Genetics and Breast Cancer

DAVID E. ANDERSON, Ph.D.

T he one clear fact that has emerged from studies of breast cancer etiology is that it is complex. This is evident in the different clinical and pathological forms of the disease, their differing rates of development, age at onset, metastatic tendencies, responses to different therapy, and survival rates. Clinical and epidemiological evidence also points to differences between patients who develop their disease premenopausally and those developing it in the postmenopausal period. Breast cancer, therefore, could be a composite of several diseases. It would then be unlikely that a single factor is the cause of all breast cancers. A variety of factors, including hormones, viruses, and genes, has already been implicated in the disease. It may well be that one or more of these factors could play a more important role in some breast cancers than in others. This report summarizes attempts at identifying those breast cancers that appear to involve a genetic component. Such identification may have utility for determining the nature of the genetic effect, whether mediated through hormones, receptor sites, or some other mechanism, and as a means by which high risk individuals may be distinguished from those at lower risk.

Interest in the possibility of a genetic basis for human breast cancer has been precipitated by the numerous pedigrees published since the nineteenth century that demonstrate familial aggregations of the disease, and by the observation that inbred strains of mice differ noticeably in their susceptibility to mammary cancer. Mouse studies have further disclosed that the action of some of the genes was localized in the physiology of hormone production by the ovaries. Other genes apparently control the response of mammary tissue to hormones; others, probably few in number, are important in the propagation and transmission of the mammary tumor virus.

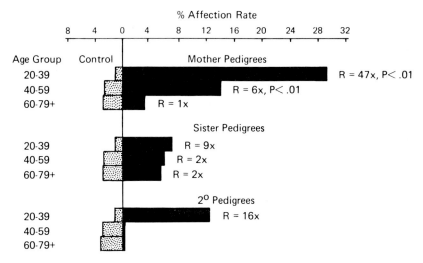

Figure 1 Percentage frequencies and risks of breast cancer in sisters of breast cancer patients compared with control sisters according to age of the sister and pedigree type.

disease in the family was confined to a sister (sister pedigrees); and (c) preexisting disease in the family involved the mother of the patient (mother pedigrees). The groups provided data for determining the risks and frequencies of breast cancer in the patients' remaining sisters (excluding those who had preexisting disease).

Extremely high risks were observed in the 84 mother pedigrees, intermediate risks in the 77 sister pedigrees, and low risks in the 73 second-degree pedigrees (Figure 1). The most striking finding was the extremely high frequency in 20- to 29 year old sisters of patients whose mothers had the disease. Approximately 30% of these sisters developed cancer, which was 47 times higher than the frequency in control sisters of the same ages. At ages 40 to 59, the risks were 6 times higher than controls, and for the oldest age group the risks were similar to control values. This decline with age was in sharp contrast to the controls where breast cancer frequency increased with age, indicating again the early occurrence of the disease in familial patients.

In the sister pedigrees, the frequency of breast cancer in the sisters at risk was threefold higher than control frequencies. The age decline in risk was not so dramatic as that in the mother pedigrees, but it was still different from that of control sisters. The findings in the second-degree pedigrees were insignificant, since only one case of breast cancer occurred in this pedigree group.

When the patients were further subdivided into those with early diagnosis and bilateral disease (Figure 2), the risks in the mother pedigrees were again highest for premenopausal sisters, approximately 33 times higher than that in premenopausal control sisters. The other pedigree groups provided no

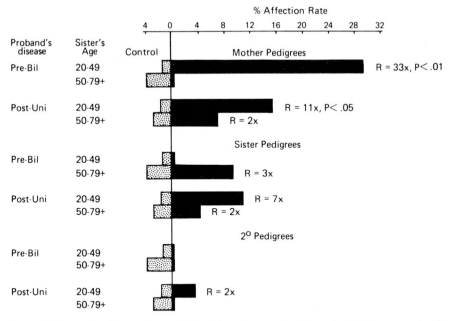

Figure 2 Percentage frequencies and risks of breast cancer in sisters of patients compared with control sisters according to age at diagnosis and laterality of the disease in the patient, age in the sister, and pedigree type.

evidence of an enhancing effect from early and bilateral disease. Obviously, the enhancing effect previously noted stemmed primarily from pedigrees where the mother of the patient had breast cancer.

This high risk group appeared to be more homogeneous than the other pedigree groups. The tumor classification was less variable (Table 2). The tumors were primarily adenocarcinomas and duct cell carcinomas, while the other pedigree groups exhibited lower frequencies of these tumors but higher frequencies of intraductal and medullary carcinomas as well as other tumor types. The variability in age at diagnosis was less ($\pm$ 1.3 years versus $\pm$ 2.5 years). Moreover, the disease frequency was highest in premenopausal sisters of patients who themselves had premenopausal disease. In fact, the correlation between age at diagnosis in the patient and her affected sisters was $r = .45$, indicating that they resembled one another more closely in age at diagnosis than did unrelated individuals. The correlation for sisters belonging to the other pedigree groups was only $r = .14$, little different from no association. In addition, the relatives in the mother pedigrees also resembled one another in developing bilateral disease. The frequency of bilaterality was 14% in the patients and 15% in their sisters. The affected mothers of bilateral patients had a higher than expected frequency of bilaterality, while among affected sisters of bilateral patients in the sister pedigrees, no such

Table 2   Tumor Classification and Other Factors According to Pedigree Type

Factor	Second-degree Pedigree	Sister Pedigree	Mother Pedigree
Tumor classification			
Adeno and duct cell carcinoma	80.8%	82.1%	91.1%
Intraductal	7.1	2.8	0.9
Medullary	1.0	6.2	1.8
Lobular	1.0	0.0	0.9
Other	7.1	6.9	2.7
Unclassified	3.0	2.1	2.7
Age at menarche (yrs.)	13.0	13.2	12.9
Age at natural menopause (yrs.)	46.8	48.0	48.4
Age at first birth (yrs.)	24.0	24.8	23.9
Nulliparity	18.0%	18.0%	21.0%
Fibrocystic disease in opposite breast	6.6%	1.3%	10.0%

excess was observed. It would thus appear that the mother pedigree category refers to a hereditary form of breast cancer (primarily adenocarcinoma and duct cell cancer) which has early onset and tends to develop as separate primaries in both breasts.

It was important to determine whether these differences in risk among the pedigree groups could be the consequence of other factors. One important consideration was other familially occurring neoplasms, which if associated with breast cancer, could influence its occurrence. One such hereditary entity has been identified and is characterized by the occurrence in close relatives of early and bilateral breast cancer in association with leukemia, brain tumor, sarcoma, and/or carcinomas of the lung, pancreas, and skin. In still another type, breast cancer may occur in association with cancer of the colon, uterus, stomach, or ovary. The pedigrees in our study group included 8 family groups considered to represent the association of breast cancer, leukemia, sarcoma, and brain tumor; and 14 families showing the association of breast, colon, uterus, stomach, or ovarian cancer. The majority of the latter group pertained to colon and/or uterine cancer, so-called hereditary adenocarcinomatosis, but these pertained solely to stomach cancer and one to ovarian cancer. These 22 cancer families accounted for only five breast cancer occurrences among sisters of patients, two in the sister and three in the mother pedigrees, all occurring in the two oldest age groups. When the 22 families were removed from the tabulations, the newly calculated risks increased slightly in the youngest age class and diminished in the two oldest classes of the mother and sister pedigrees compared with Figure 1. Consequently, these cancer families, which could have influenced the familial frequency of breast cancer, apparently had little influence on the differences in risk observed among the pedigree groups.

The occurrence of these families serves to indicate that there may be several types of hereditary breast cancer: an early, bilateral, site specific type, as observed in the mother pedigrees; an early, bilateral type associated primarily with leukemia, sarcoma, and brain tumors; and a later occurring, more unilateral type occurring in association with colon and uterine cancer. Another type may also be associated with stomach cancer, as observed in 3 of the present families; and another with ovarian cancer, as observed in one family in this group and previously in 3 of 34 families. The sister pedigrees could refer to a heterogeneous and less heritable group with a threefold increased risk for sisters and where the first disease tends to be late occurring and unilateral.

Other factors long implicated in breast cancer, such as age at menarche, menopause, first birth, or nulliparity and parity, were also evaluated, but no significant differences were observed among the pedigree groups. Fibrocystic disease in the opposite breast of a patient with breast cancer was more frequent than expected in the mother pedigrees, assuming fibrocystic disease to occur independently of pedigree type. No attempt has yet been made to determine whether fibrocystic disease is also more frequent in the breast harboring the cancerous lesions. Haagensen considered gross cystic disease to be familial and to increase the risk of cancer development. Moreover, benign lesions of the breast, including cystic disease, are more frequent in premenopausal than postmenopausal women. This finding, among others, led de Waard to propose that ovarian estrogens play an important role in premenopausal breast cancer. Since the genetic effect is strongest in premenopausal patients, then conceivably the genetic effect could be associated with ovarian activity. Corroboration for this possibility was provided by the mother pedigrees, where the frequencies and risks were highest during the period of highest ovarian activity, declined in the period of decreasing ovarian activity, and were lowest in the menopausal period when the ovaries are largely nonfunctional.

The possibility of ovarian involvement could have relevance to the proposal of Lemon that there may be a genetic basis for the hydroxylation of estrone and 17-beta-estradiol to estriol. He postulated a mutant gene that reduces 16-alpha-hydroxylase activity, which in turn results in reduction of the ratio of urinary estriol/estrone + 17-beta-estradiol. Since estriol may be protective against breast cancer, a reduction in this hormone could be associated with an increased risk. This is an attractive proposal and should be pursued. It might offer a means for identifying individuals at high risk to breast cancer.

How a genetic etiologic component for breast cancer might relate to a viral agent is also of interest. Viral particles have been observed in the milk of a significant fraction of women with family histories of breast cancer and homology has been shown between the base sequences of RNA molecules from extracts of human breast cancer tissue and the RNA of the Bittner mouse mammary tumor virus. If a virus were involved in breast cancer, higher frequencies of the disease would be expected in the maternal side of a family than in the paternal side. This type of comparison was possible in the present data. Regardless of the type of comparison, no significant differences were observed. In fact, the frequencies in grandmothers and aunts were similar and averaged 15.3% in paternal relatives compared with 10.6% in maternal relatives. Both were higher than the 2.7% in controls. Among the sisters of patients whose grandmothers had breast cancer, those with a paternal lineage exhibited a 3% frequency of the disease and those with a maternal lineage, 3.8%. This difference is not significant nor is either value significantly different from the controls. These comparisons thus indicate that males may well be involved in the transmission of breast cancer and that there is no higher disease frequency in maternal lineages. This would argue against the cytoplasmic or milk transmission of a virus but not against the possible transmission of viral information integrated into the host's DNA.

The possibility of a milk transmitted virus was also evaluated through another approach. If an agent were transmitted through milk, its effect would be more evident in the mother pedigrees than in the others, because all of the mothers in this pedigree group had the disease and their daughters had a significantly higher disease frequency, while the mothers in the other pedigree groups were unaffected and their daughters had low frequencies of the disease. Breast feeding should thus have played a more important role in the mother pedigrees than in the others. No such difference was found (Figure 3). There was little or no difference among the pedigree groups in the numbers of patients who were breast fed or in the duration of their breast feeding. Consequently, neither a cytoplasmic nor a milk transmitted virus appeared to be involved; or if one were involved, it was ubiquitous.

Before advising a woman of her risk of developing breast cancer, attention should be given to (a) her age, (b) the age at diagnosis and laterality of the disease in her mother and/or sister, and (c) the pattern of breast cancer in her family, particularly the status of her mother and/or her sisters. Family histories should also include digestive and genital neoplasms, leukemia, sarcoma, and brain tumors. Women at increased risk should be screened regularly by mammography and physical examination. In the present study, about 30% of the sisters of patients with family histories of the disease had at least a 3.5 times increased risk of breast cancer, and approximately 40% of these or 12% of the total were in the extremely high risk group. The early age at occurrence of cancer indicates that screening examinations should not be postponed until 35 or 40 years of age as is now sometimes recommended, but should be instituted at an early age whenever a genetically high risk

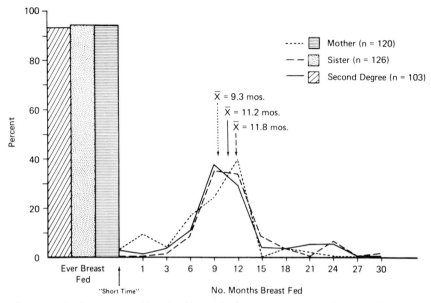

Figure 3 The frequency and length of breast feeding in patients according to pedigree type.

woman is identified. It is generally accepted that women should be examined at yearly intervals, but in view of the rapid development of carcinoma in high risk families, this concept should perhaps be replaced by a more individualized program of surveillance. A program of periodic examination for genetically high risk women, even at relatively young ages, should result in the detection of breast lesions at an earlier stage and one more amenable to treatment.

Defining the Problem: A Panel Discussion

Moderator: BENJAMIN F. BYRD, Jr., M.D.
THOMAS CARLILE, M.D.
ROBERT L. EGAN, M.D.
LAMAN A. GRAY, M.D.
JUSTIN J. STEIN, M.D.
JOHN D. WALLACE
ASHBEL C. WILLIAMS, M.D.

DR. BYRD: Dr Carlile, what effect does the use of estrogens or the pill have on mammography?

DR. CARLILE: I have no substantial information, either from our own experience or that of others, that there is any change that can be demonstrated in mammograms of people who are on hormones.

DR. GRAY: Modern birth control pills, with their very low estrogen and low progesterone content, produce little clinical effect on the average breast. The only changes are intermittent swelling, congestion, and nodularity. The mammographic changes are the same as those of early pregnancy.

DR. EGAN: When the pill first became rampant, I reviewed a series of mammograms from patients with known histories of taking these drugs but could not differentiate with any certainty at all which were on the pill and which were not.

DR. BYRD: Mr. Wallace, what about the effects of estrogens on thermography?

MR. WALLACE: The mean temperature of both breasts is increased in patients taking the pill, but the venous patterns and so forth are unaltered. Oral contraceptives do not interfere with thermographic diagnosis.

DR. BYRD: Are there any questions from the floor?

QUESTION: Dr. Carlile, is there a mammography unit available that would allow me to use a tungsten anode in the low kV range, or do I have to go to a molybdenum anode tube to accomplish this?

DR. CARLILE: A number of the manufacturers offer the option of either a tungsten or molybdenum anode tube in units made specifically for doing mammograms in the upright position. This is already available.

QUESTION: Should mammographic examination be restricted to women over 25?

DR. CARLILE: There are two factors involved in that question. The first is that mammography is less accurate under the age of 40. Second, with the imprecise state of knowledge about dosimetry in mammography, we prefer not to irradiate women in the childbearing age. In the breast cancer screening centers, the minimal age is 35, and this is realistic for survey purposes. Of course, we do mammography in women under 35 who have symptoms or signs of breast disease.

QUESTION: Is it permissible to continue Premarin or other estrogens in postmenopausal women who have duct hyperplasia or papillomas?

DR. GRAY: I don't think so. We do not think that estrogens cause cancer, but once cancer is formed, 30% are estrogen dependent. Since there is a high possibility of concomitant cancer in a patient with findings of this sort, estrogens, which might make the cancer grow more rapidly, are to be avoided.

DR. WILLIAMS: I concur completely with what Dr. Gray has said.

DR. BYRD: Dr. Egan, in your long experience you have identified many occult cancers. Have you ever had difficulty in getting surgeons to operate on the basis of mammographic findings alone?

DR. EGAN: At first, even at Anderson Hospital, no one would operate on a cancer found by mammography only. Acceptance has been a gradual process. This has been true both in my own case and around the United States.

DR. CARLILE: Our experience has been the same as Dr. Egan's. Once you demonstrate to a surgeon that you can detect a cancer he cannot palpate, he becomes much more enthusiastic about mammography.

DR. EGAN: There is a syndrome I have found commonly among surgeons. For example, Dr. Sam Wilkins, with whom I work now, often says, "Boy, I can really feel those things after you localize them for me!"

DR. BYRD: I suppose that is what is known as the "educated touch."

DR. WILLIAMS: To return to the earlier question about age limits for mammography, we have had in our detection program a tumor detected by mammography in a patient 23 years of age. Dr. McClow thought the mass was cancer, but the surgeon could not feel it. He was so sure of his physical findings that he did the biopsy without being prepared to do a radical. Subsequently, when the presence of cancer was histologically confirmed, he had the embarrassing experience of having to tell the patient and having to go back and do the mastectomy several days later. In general, however, our age indications are the same as those that have been stipulated. We do not do mammography under 35 years of age unless there is a specific problem.

DR. G. F. ROBBINS: I would like to ask Dr. Gray if he believes that the problem of phlebitis and embolism is serious enough that the use of birth control pills should be limited?

DR. GRAY: Although phlebitis can be serious, it is a lot less serious than the complication of pregnancy. At least, I think so. As a matter of fact, the incidence of thrombophlebitis has always been low and it is even less with the newer preparations. I have not seen a single case among several thousand patients in the past three years.

QUESTION: Greenblatt and others have written that progesterone can be given to reduce cystic hyperplasia of breasts. If this is the case, can progesterone be given for the control of menopausal symptoms in patients with papillomas and duct hyperplasia?

DR. GRAY: I believe that progesterone is a causative factor in fibrocystic disease. If a patient had much hyperplasia and much hyperactivty of mammary tissue, I would not use any hormonal therapy.

QUESTION: I would like to report a case of my own similar to Dr. Williams'. A 22 year old woman was referred with a huge hard mass in one breast, clinically considered to be a giant fibroadenoma. On mammography, at the apex of the tumor there were seen a few tiny microcalcifications. At surgery, the large mass was found to be benign, but there was also a carcinoma exactly at the location shown radiographically. This experience brings up a question: Is it advisable to do mammography on a regular basis in women in the childbearing age with heavy nodular breasts?

DR. CARLILE: Based upon family history, the patient's degree of concern, the symptomatology and the physical findings, it might be appropriate to schedule mammography at some selected interval. This might be less frequently than for older women, say, every two years or even three years. I think it is also critically important that such a patient should learn self-examination and report to her physician if she observes any change at all. Mammography in this situation should be used judiciously and not as an automatic routine.

DR. EGAN: I think mammography has important applications at any age. For example, among women under 32 who have a palpable nodule but no visible mass in the mammogram, less than 1 in 40 will prove to have cancer.

Mammography added to clinical examination can give a great deal of confidence that a suspect lesion is not cancer and then, biopsy can be done electively.

DR. BYRD: As one might have anticipated, this very interesting discussion is being terminated by lack of time rather than by lack of interest. Thank you members of the panel and audience for your participation.

PART TWO

MAMMOGRAPHY AND
THE SYMPTOMATIC BREAST

The Physician, the Lump, and the Mammogram

CHARLES W. HAYDEN, M.D.

To the physician faced with the ever increasing problem of the woman with a lump in her breast, there are three important sources of data: the patient, the physician himself, and the mammogram. To achieve optimal results, certain conditions are necessary in each of these. The patient, still the best detector of tumors, must be dedicated to breast self-examination. We encourage using soapy fingers at the time of each bath in addition to the recommended monthly procedure outlined by the American Cancer Society. She should also know her own risk factor and be prepared, whenever indicated, to seek breast examination by her physician, surgeon, or gynecologist. From physicians, we ask a high index of suspicion for breast cancer, careful history taking, identification of high risk patients, and thorough breast examinations. This last should be a part of each physical examination of a woman, regardless of her complaint. From the mammogram, with experience, we have come to anticipate both benefits and shortcomings. All agree that mammography is inferior to physical examination in young women with dense glandular breasts. On the other hand, mammography is superior to physical examination in large pendulous breasts, since it can detect tumors that are not palpable.

To obtain the best of all three of these worlds, it is necessary to individualize the approach to the patient with breast complaints, from the minute she walks into the office, through detection and diagnosis, through decision as to type of treatment, and into the period of follow-up. I would like to focus on four areas in which mammography plays a role in this individualization. These are are the following:

1. Defining guidelines and ground rules for using mammography.
2. Capitalizing on the by-products of mammography.
3. Defining the value of mammography in the second breast problem.
4. The value of the specimen mammogram.

The guidelines and basic ground rules that we are using for mammography are as follows:

1. We expect the radiologist to select the technique that gives the best possible images with the least radiation risk to our patients, and to achieve an accuracy of 90%.
2. The mammogram should never be used in place of a biopsy when a dominant lesion is present, but rather as an adjunct and as a base line screen for the opposite breast.
3. The mammogram should never change the basic surgical approach in breast disease. A lump is a lump, and it must be biopsied either by the needle or the knife. Too often when dealing with a mass a surgeon may say, "Why do I need a mammogram? I know what to do." Unfortunately, he forgets about multicentricity, bilaterality, and the risk of in situ carcinoma.
4. In order to achieve the 90% accuracy expectation, it is necessary for the radiologist to do a physical examination of the breast in conjunction with the mammogram.
5. To individualize the use of the mammogram, patients should be grouped according to their breast complaints and clinical findings. Group A patients are those with dominant lesions or lumps. Here mammography is strictly a complementary or adjunctive procedure and must never be used in place of surgery. Group B patients are those with complaints or symptoms referable to the breast but who do not have dominant lesions or masses. The mammogram helps to distinguish true masses from false ones and helps in characterizing indefinite areas of thickening. If nothing distinctive is seen on the mammogram and if careful, frequent clinical examinations reveal nothing, a conservative course is justified. If, on the other hand, the patient is in a high risk group, and especially if she has had a previous breast cancer, any suspicious area must be biopsied early and not followed. Group C patients are those without complaints or clinical findings but who are in the high risk population. Here mammography is essentially a screening procedure.

To obtain the best of the world of mammography we capitalize on its by-products (see Table 1) which are as follows:

Table 1   Surgical By-Products of Mammography

1. Finding occult carcinoma.
2. Demonstrating tumors when small; less node involvement.
3. Pre-operative screening of opposite breast.
4. Post-mastectomy examinations aid in earlier tumor detection.
5. Prevents repeated biopsies in fibrocystic disease.
6. Aids in examination of large pendulous breasts.
7. Improves accuracy of pre-operative diagnosis.
8. Aids in O.R. scheduling.
9. Screening of high risk patients.
10. Brings patients for examination and operation earlier.
11. Improves knowledge of breast diseases and gives new and objective approach to differential diagnosis.

1. Finding occult carcinomas.
2. Demonstrating tumors when they are small and less likely to have node involvement. This has been a distinct advance at our hospital. Pathological Stage 2 patients have dropped from 55.6% in the premammography era to 36.5% at present.
3. Preoperative screening of the opposite breast. This is necessary as a base for comparisons with future studies during the follow-up period.
4. Detection of cancer in the remaining breast before it becomes palpable.
5. Prevention of repeated biopsies in fibrocytic disease.
6. Examination of large pendulous breasts, one source of occult tumors.
7. Improvement in the accuracy of preoperative diagnosis.
8. Assistance in operating room scheduling.
9. Screening of high risk patients. (See Table 2.)
10. Improvement in the knowledge of breast disease among the physician population.

Table 2   High Risk Patients

1. Never married
2. Nulliparous
3. No lactation
4. Family history of cancer
5. Previous breast surgery
6. Previous pelvic surgery
7. Hormone therapy

An additional by-product of mammography is its help in clinical staging. Staging has always been fraught with inaccuracies. Gold et al. in 1972 reported that, in a study of 58 women who had radical mastectomies for infiltrating duct carcinoma, the extent of local tumor as recorded by mammography correlated with the frequency of concomitant metastases to the axillary lymph nodes. They classified the tumors into highly infiltrative (scirrhous, spiculate, stellate) or slightly infiltrative (circumscribed, knobby). Positive axillary nodes were found in 58% of the highly infiltrative tumors but in only 21% of the slightly infiltrative tumors.

The multidisciplinary approach to decision making is part of the changing pattern of breast cancer therapy. Prognostic determination and staging are based on clinical, radiographic, surgical, and pathological findings. The integration of these evaluations gives a clue to the potential of a particular tumor in an individual patient and thereby guides therapy in accordance with her biological needs. Mammography has an important role in this approach.

Stewart and Foote first called attention to the problem of the second breast with the statement that the most frequent precancerous lesion of the breast is a cancer of the opposite breast (Table 3). It was not until the report of Urban on his random biopsies of opposite breasts and that of Leis on his findings in selective prophylactic simple mastectomies that the real magnitude of the problem became evident. Both reports showed a much higher incidence of simultaneous and nonsimultaneous cancers than had ever been expected (Table 4). The high incidence of lobular carcinoma in situ in both series underscores the importance of mammography, since this earliest of early cancers has few, if any, clinical manifestations.

To individualize our approach to the opposite breast after mastectomy for carcinoma we use the following procedures:

1. Careful periodic physical examinations every three months for two years and every six months thereafter.

Table 3   Bilateral Breast Carcinoma

F. STEWART & F. FOOTE:
"The female breast is a precancerous organ and the most frequent precancerous lesion of the breast is a cancer of the opposite breast."

J.A. URBAN:
"There is an increasing awareness of the bilaterality of breast cancer. The same factors that cause the development of a cancer of one breast are capable of affecting the appearance of a similar lesion in the opposite breast."

D.P. Slaughter:
"...the breasts represent a single system and would predictabley become affected bilaterally."

Table 4   Bilateral Breast Carcinoma

	Method	Cases	Ca	% Bilateral
Leis, H.P., Jr. 1967	Prophylactic Opposite Mastectomy	71	11	15.5% 6 Ca in-situ 5 infiltrating Ca (7%)
Urban, J.A.	Simultaneous biopsy opposite breast	159	31	19.5% 18 Ca in-situ 13 infiltrating Ca (8%)
Missakian, M et al, 1965	Post-mastectomy follow-up mammography	397	25	6%

2. Mammography annually or more often if indicated.
3. Early biopsy of clinically or mammographically suspicious area.
4. Blind random biopsy of the upper outer quadrant and mirror image areas in high risk patients.
5. Prophylactic total mastectomy in selected high risk patients.

We have used specimen mammography when confronted with the need to biopsy a nonpalatable density found on mammogram. This need is occurring more often as emphasis shifts to the search for occult and minimal cancers. Not only patterns of calcification, but also new soft tissue densities appearing in serial mammograms may be involved.

In brief, our procedure is to take an adequate excisional biopsy, usually a quadrant of the breast. The specimen is x-rayed prior to sectioning to assure the surgeon that he has removed the correct area. The radiologist indicates the site for histologic sampling by comparing the preoperative and specimen mammograms. We have not insisted on frozen section of these dubious areas, being content to wait for paraffin sections in order to have the most accurate information possible. The risk of a brief delay between biopsy and definite surgery is negligible. The yield from this procedure has been well worth the extra effort, especially in solving the problem of a suspicious area seen in a remaining breast.

These are the things I wish I could say to every young surgeon concerned with the proper approach to the management of breast cancer. Learn to use all your sources of information. Encourage careful self-examination. Sympathetically check the patient's findings. If she feels something, believe her. Be diligent and thorough about breast examinations. Seek out high risk patients by good history taking. Do repeated mammograms in high risk patients. Biopsy dominant and suspicious areas early. Shorten the interval between examinations in high risk patients. Don't be complacent about a

present. We do not do a bone survey on all patients. If there is bone pain, or if operability is borderline, we do. But in 10 years only 19% of our operable patients developed bone metastases, so we feel that routine bone survey should not be done. I think too that it is very important to explain in detail to patients what they can anticipate. They need to know, for example, why partial mastectomy is not valid treatment. This takes time, but the results are worth it.

DR. TAYLOR: Dr. Powell, do you think all dominant nodules should be biopsied?

DR. POWELL: They should all be diagnosed. Formal biopsy is only one method of doing this. Another is observation, particularly in the patient with lumpy breasts after she has a menstrual period. Frequently a biopsy can be avoided this way. A third means, of course, is aspiration of a cyst for diagnosis.

DR. TAYLOR: How do you feel about following a patient who has a palpable nodule which is considered radiographically to look benign? Is that ever a problem?

DR. ROBBINS: We do not adopt that procedure very often. Anybody who follows a dominant mass by mammography indefinitely without at least using a needle to find out whether it is a cyst is asking for a lawsuit.

DR. TAYLOR: Dr. Gold, would you comment on the role of mammography in the symptomatic patient?

DR. GOLD: The role of mammography in the symptomatic patient should be recognized as being limited. It is true that mammographic evaluation of a mass may permit better planning of the surgical procedure or that it may give some assurance to the patient of the probable benignity of the mass. But mammography cannot be depended upon invariably to evaluate a mass correctly. Most benign masses are well-circumscribed and appear so mammographically, and most malignant masses have spiculated or indistinct margins, but benign masses may simulate malignant ones in mammograms and vice versa. Moreover, in a radiographically dense breast, a palpable mass can be completely masked. Characteristic calcifications can be detected in one-third to one-half of breast cancers, but identical calcifications may be seen in benign disorders such as papillomatosis and sclerosing adenosis.

Because of these considerations, any dominant mass in a woman over the age of 30 should be biopsied, or an attempt should be made at aspiration, no matter what the mammographic features. By the same token, a nonpalpable but radiographically suspicious area should be biopsied even in the absence of a palpable mass. The primary purpose of mammography in the symptomatic patient is not so much the evaluation of the palpable mass but rather the evaluation of both breasts for signs of occult cancer in other areas. If suspicious findings are detected, a biopsy of that area can be performed at the same time the palpable mass is excised. Breast cancer is simultaneously bilateral in 5% of patients and signs of bilaterality should be sought, especially in women who have a history of breast cancer on the maternal side of the family.

DR. TAYLOR: Dr. Robbins, do you order a mammogram on every patient with a nodule?

DR. ROBBINS: On all of those in whom we suspect cancer, we do. On the young girls with nodules we are pretty sure are fibroadenomas, we do not. We are, all of us, ordering a lot of mammograms.

DR. TAYLOR: Dr. Powell, what about symptoms of pain or tenderness? Are these reassuring, or do you disregard them?

DR. POWELL: I generally disregard them. Only 15 to 20% of cancers are painful or tender. Severe tenderness almost always indicates benign disease. As a general rule, pain and tenderness should not influence a decision for management.

DR. TAYLOR: What about the patient who has lumpy breasts or multiple masses? Do you modify your approach to these people?

DR. POWELL: We do mammography as a base line on lumpy breasts and, of course, we check them after a menstrual period. If one area seems to be firmer or in some other way more suspect, we do a biopsy. If the biopsy diagnosis is benign, we follow the patient very closely, much more closely than the average patient, and also teach and encourage periodic self-examination.

DR. ROBBINS: What Dr. Powell says makes a lot of sense. We follow the same line. The lumpy breast premenstrually is just uninterpretable. They should be reexamined postmenstrually.

DR. TAYLOR: Let us get down to the matter of the biopsy and discuss it for a bit. Dr. Robbins, do you appreciate a radiologist's telling you something should be aspirated or biopsied?

DR. ROBBINS: I would be a damn fool if I didn't. In the past I have made mistakes this way. It is an absolute necessity to have three people involved: the surgeon, the radiologist, and the pathologist. As for aspiration biopsy, you have to be somewhat sadistic to get an adequate specimen and you have to have a cytologist who is doing a lot of aspiration biopsy studies. If you have that team, aspiration saves time in the operating room and makes it a little easier to plan the surgery.

Excisional biopsy is fine for a big lump. We do a generous excision, practically a quadrant, because all too often we have found small cancers that could not be detected, even by mammography, in the area of a benign dominant mass. The important thing is the team work and getting enough tissue so the pathologist can make a reasonably accurate diagnosis.

DR. ROSEN: Let me amplify what Dr. Robbins has said. In any institution, one has to make the most of the aptitudes of the people available. If there is someone who is interested and expert in cytology, that is something to be used. For the average pathologist who sees relatively little material, aspiration cytology is probably not advisable. A better shortcut is the plug needle biopsy. This should be used for establishing the diagnosis when the clinical setting is strongly suggestive of carcinoma. In the situation of the ill-defined mass, excisional biopsy is indicated as Dr. Robbins pointed out, because one frequently finds something in an area where one did not expect to find it. For exploratory biopsies, excisional biopsy is best. Needle biopsy or needle aspiration should be reserved for lesions almost certain to be carcinoma.

DR. TAYLOR: Dr. Bauermeister, do you agree with this? Is the office biopsy of breast nodules desirable? Are there other alternatives?

DR. BAUERMEISTER: I agree that in the hands of an expert, aspiration cytology is an excellent procedure, but most practicing pathologists find it difficult to interpret. Plug needle biopsy, however, is comparatively easy. Our surgeons use a needle similar to that used for liver biopsies. They obtain a nice core of tissue. With current frozen section techniques, good sections can be obtained and a reliable diagnosis can be rendered in most situations. Most pathologists should be able to handle the core biopsy if the procedure is reserved for lesions clinically almost surely cancer. This can be done as an outpatient procedure or in the operating room in lieu of an open biopsy. Either way it saves operating room time.

DR. ROBBINS: Everyone should realize that a negative needle biopsy doesn't mean anything and certainly should be followed by another biopsy.

DR. ROSEN: That emphasizes the point that needle biopsy should be reserved for the mass almost sure to be carcinoma. A negative result should be followed by operative biopsy. I should like also to say something about cyst aspiration while we're talking about cytology. If the cyst fluid is bloody, or if there is a mass near the cyst which remains after the cyst is evacuated, there may be some value in doing cytologic examination of the fluid. The vast majority of cysts, however, will produce negative results. There is very little need for cytologic examination when the fluid is clear. There are studies in process concerning biochemical analysis of cyst fluids, and in the future this may prove to be of prognostic importance.

DR. BAUERMEISTER: A previous question was concerned with excisional biopsy done as an outpatient procedure. In our experience this has resulted in significant morbidity. The biopsy is often limited. I think excisional biopsy should be an operating room procedure.

DR. ROBBINS: I understand that Dr. Loren Humphrey is carrying out a study on this at the University of Kansas in Kansas City, but nothing has been published about it yet. I have occasionally done an excision in the office in the case of a girl with an obvious fibroadenoma. If she doesn't have insurance, the economics of it make sense. I certainly have an open mind on the subject.

DR. BAUERMEISTER: We have been handling biopsy patients on an in-and-out basis. The patient is admitted the morning of surgery and a bed is reserved for her. The surgery is scheduled for mid-morning. A frozen section is done on the biopsy specimen. If it is benign, the bed reservation is then canceled, and the patient receives no bed or room charge. She is discharged that afternoon from the recovery room. This saves the patient $150.00 to $200.00, since she is not actually admitted before the operation.

DR. TAYLOR: Dr. Rosen, do you do specimen radiography as a routine? How do you set up the mechanism for it?

DR. ROSEN: Because of experiences with poor coordination, we have adopted a policy of scheduling specimen radiography on the operating schedule, just as one would schedule an operative cholangiogram or other radiologic procedure during the course of surgery. By doing this we have introduced a certain amount of discipline which alerts all of the people who have to participate in the procedure. This is definitely a multidisciplinary activity. It involves the surgeon, the pathologist, and frequently a radiologist as well. It is important to have some scheduling of these kinds of cases. Specimen radiography is done at the time of surgery only if there is a suspicious mammogram and no palpable mass. Roentgenographic studies of other specimens are done after surgery is completed.

DR. TAYLOR: Dr. Robbins, do you find any problem in communicating with your radiologist or your pathologist?

DR. ROBBINS: No, we do not. We are very fortunate in having a group that works together well. We include these people in our conferences. I think it is important to be friendly and work with them all the time and not just when you have difficulties.

DR. BAUERMEISTER: Since we are talking about communication, it might be well to point out that if the lesion is occult and the surgeon is faced with the blind biopsy problem, it is essential that he communicate with the radiologist who has read the mammogram, preferably personally looking at the films as a team, so they can localize the area to be biopsied.

DR. TAYLOR: Dr. Gold, as you follow patients who have had multiple biopsies, is this a problem? Do you sometimes give false positive readings or mislead your surgeons?

DR. GOLD: We make physical examination of the breast and axilla a regular practice in all of our patients. We have a diagram of the breasts on which we record the locations of scars from previous biopsies. We take this into account when we interpret the mammogram. If the mammographer does not see the patient, he has no idea where these scars are, and he may encounter difficulty in interpretation. Retraction is often associated with scars, particularly if they result from quadrant resections. This can simulate carcinoma.

DR. ROSEN: I would like to go back to something about cytology. We did not touch on the problem of nipple secretions. In our experience, when there is a spontaneous discharge from the breast, cytology may be useful, especially if the fluid is bloody. If the result is negative, this should not be taken as final, but the patient should be fully evaluated with mammography and obviously with physical examination for the possibility of an occult lesion.

FROM THE FLOOR: I would like to present a point. What has been said about coordination and team effort is all very well and nobody can disagree. But the vast majority of breast cancers are not diagnosed or treated at Memorial Hospital. They are diagnosed in a busy family physician's office. They are referred to a private radiologist who does mammography. Then they are referred to a surgeon who examines the lump in his office and admits the individual to a hospital, using the information that has been gathered in three or four different places. This is how it is done, whether it is desirable or not. We need to work toward standardization of procedures and of terminology, as well as topographical, radiologic description of masses. This would make this type of operation more successful than it is now.

DR. TAYLOR: I believe he has raised a point that may not be answerable. Dr. Powell, would you comment, please?

DR. POWELL: Regardless of the size of the hospital or any other consideration, cooperation and coordination between radiologist and surgeon is essential. If you do not have that, mammography isn't worthwhile. Under those circumstances, I would just as soon make decisions on the basis of clinical grounds alone.

DR. TAYLOR: I regret that our time has expired. I want to thank the panelists for their participation and the audience for its interest.

Evaluation of Nipple Discharge

HENRY P. LEIS, Jr., M.D.

Next to a lump in the breast, nipple discharge is the most common complaint of women admitted to the hospital for breast surgery. About 7% of patients with breast lesions have nipple discharge. It occurs in about 10% of women with benign lesions and in 3% of those with malignancies. In the male, it has a more serious prognostic import, occurring in 15–20% of male breast cancers.

In a series of 3287 breast operations at New York Medical College and Affiliated Hospitals during the 10 year period 1960–1969, there were 259 patients (7.8% of the total) who had nipple discharge. Of the 2367 with benign lesions, 230 or 9.7% had nipple discharge and of the 923 with malignant lesions, 29 or 3.1% had discharge.

There are seven basic types of discharge:

1. Milky, due to galactorrhea
2. Sticky (grumous), multicolored, due to duct ectasia
3. Purulent, due to infection
4. Watery
5. Serous
6. Serosanguineous
7. Bloody

The serous, serosanguineous, and bloody discharges are the most common types among patients hospitalized for surgery. These and the rare watery discharge are also the most important, since they may be due to cancer. In decreasing order of frequency, these types of discharge are due to intraduc-

69

tal papilloma, fibrocystic disease, cancer, and advanced duct ectasia (plasma cell mastitis). They may also occur in marked engorgement due to pregnancy. Over the age of 50, however, cancer is the leading cause of these types of discharge.

Many discharges are due to benign lesions and can be treated medically. Since, however, a discharge may herald a malignant lesion, each patient should be carefully investigated. In general, only spontaneous discharges have pathologic significance, but recently Sartorius has emphasized the possible value of stimulating discharges from asymptomatic women as a means of detecting unsuspected cancer. He uses a special suction device.

Classification of a discharge into one of the seven basic types can usually be accomplished by observation of its color and consistency, by palpation to determine if it is sticky, and by staining with Wright's stain to determine the presence or absence of pus or blood. A drop placed on a white sponge produces a reddish color with lighter shadings of red extending to the periphery if blood is present.

If the discharge is due to cancer, a mass is usually palpable, but this is not always true. Cytology is a valuable aid but it is unsafe to rely on it to determine the presence or absence of a cancer, since the percentage of false negatives is quite high. An accuracy of about 80% can be expected. Greatest accuracy is obtained by careful preparation of the smear, as outlined by Frost, and by diligent examination by a highly trained cytologist.

Mammography is also valuable in differentiating between benign and malignant lesions, but its accuracy is only about 85%. Contrast mammography, as outlined by Funderburk and Syphax, is more valuable than soft tissue mammography in the diagnosis and localization of intraductal papillomas.

Galactorrhea, a milky discharge, is usually persistent postpartum lactation. It also occurs in certain endocrine disorders accompanied by amenorrhea, and in patients under treatment with oral contraceptives and certain tranquilizers. It is caused by an increased production of prolactin and is treated medically by stopping any etiologic agent, by large doses of estrogen to suppress the pituitary, by the administration of progesterone to inhibit prolactin, or by giving clomiphene citrate to stimulate the hypothalamus.

Duct ectasia or comedomastitis usually occurs in women near the menopause and produces a multicolored, sticky (grumous) discharge with burning and itching of the nipple and areola. If the disease progresses, inflammatory changes and subsequent fibrosis result in the formation of a mass that can mimic cancer. This stage is called plasma cell mastitis. If a mass is present, surgical excision should be done, but otherwise medical therapy with Phisohex or Betadine nipple hygiene, avoidance of all nipple manipulation, and in some cases the administration of estrogens is usually adequate.

Acute puerperal mastitis, chronic lactation mastitis, and central abscesses produce purulent discharges. Appropriate antibiotic therapy is sometimes effective but if suppuration occurs, incisional drainage is needed.

Although the rare watery discharge and the more common serous, serosanguineous, and bloody discharges are usually due to benign lesions, they can also be due to cancer and therefore demand surgical exploration. Even the absence of a palpable mass, negative cytology, and a negative mammography cannot be regarded as excluding the possibility of carcinoma. Furthermore, lesions such as intraductal papillomas and papillary epithelial hyperplasia with atypia, a form of fibrocytic disease, may be premalignant and should be removed.

We believe that the most suitable surgical procedure in this situation is complete excision of the central ducts through a periareolar incision. With care, good cosmetic results can be obtained. In women under 30 and in those anxious to have children, occasionally it is better to excise only the clinically involved duct with a wedge of adjacent breast tissue. Usually it is best to rely on a permanent paraffin section rather than a frozen section, since it may be difficult to differentiate premalignant lesions with atypia from in situ carcinoma.

Contrast Mammography

DAVID D. PAULUS, M.D.

Contrast mammography, the contrast injection of the ductal systems of the breast, is a safe and simple radiographic procedure involving minimal discomfort to the patient. It can clarify the anatomy of a discharging duct system and precisely locate intraductal pathology.

The technique is simple. A plain mammogram is obtained immediately before injection. The patient is placed in comfortable supine position on the x-ray table, and the breast gently palpated by radial stroking to locate the ostium of the discharging duct system. It is imperative that an actively discharging duct be present. Without a discharge, it is impossible to locate the offending duct, and almost impossible to cannulate an ostium.

The nipple, areola, and surrounding skin are cleansed with Betadine and alcohol. With a rounded smooth probe, the nipple is gently explored at the site of the discharge to locate the ostium of the involved duct. The duct is then cannulated with a blunt 25 or 26 gauge needle.

Injection is done slowly until the patient experiences a feeling of fullness. This requires 0.5 to 2 ml. The contrast medium used is water soluble, the same one used for intravenous pyelography. The patient is asked to indicate the area where she feels a sensation of fullness as the medium is injected and to say when slight burning is felt.

This is the end point of the injection. The needle is withdrawn and the patient is immediately positioned for the lateral and craniocaudal mammographic projections. The images are processed and reviewed immediately.

Although contrast mammography is not new, there are only a few reported series in the literature. Funderburk has described studies involving 36 breasts, almost two-thirds of which showed bloody or serous discharge. The majority proved to have intraductal papilloma or papillomatosis. In a series of 75 cases reported by Rummel, the most frequent diagnoses were, as might be expected, duct ectasia or periductal mastitis and intraductal papilloma. There were 8 cases of carcinoma, surprisingly. One of these was clinically palpable and 2 had positive mammograms. The remaining 6 were demonstrated by the contrast study only. The 21 cases reported by Nunnerly and Field in 1972 included 6 cases of papilloma, 8 cases of duct ectasia, and 2 cases with dilated subareolar ducts, similar to those in papilloma, but without filling defects. There was 1 carcinoma demonstrated by plain mammogram in which dilated, distorted ducts were present.

The most recently reported series, that of Thereat and Appelman, involved 54 injections. Eighteen were normal, there was ectasia in 27, papillomas in 14, ductal masses, probably papillomas, in 17. There were 2 cases of carcinoma. Both patients had bloody discharges. One had a palpable mass, and both showed irregular, poorly filled ducts.

Contrast mammography is superior to any other single procedure in determining the cause of nipple discharge prior to surgery.

Intraductal papilloma is the most common cause of a bloody nipple discharge. There is an increased incidence of cancer in patients with intraductal papilloma, suggesting that it is a premalignant lesion.

A negative contrast mammogram should not exclude other diagnostic procedures. In benign disease, contrast mammography can justify performance of a limited resection of the involved area, result in providing only pertinent tissue for the pathologist, and preserve normal, unaffected tissue with obvious cosmetic advantages.

Histologic Patterns
of Breast Cancer with
Special Significance

HERBERT B. TAYLOR, M.D.

Although we refer to breast cancer as if it were a single entity, it is actually a disease with many histologic variations, differing in their natural histories, clinical behavior, and prognosis. In comparative studies, these variations must be taken into consideration. While a majority of breast cancers in any series are of the common infiltrating duct type, a minority will be kinds that have significantly more favorable prognoses and the percentage of these included in any study will affect the survival statistics.

Of the several types of mammary cancer having more favorable prognoses, all are rare in this country but somewhat more frequent in other countries. They constitute perhaps one-sixth of all mammary cancers.

One of this group is the adenoid cystic carcinoma of the breast. It usually forms a well-circumscribed, small discrete nodule, difficult to delineate from the adjacent mammary tissue. The histologic pattern consists of cystic spaces, surrounded by small cells, and is similar to adenoid cystic carcinomas occurring in other parts of the body. Those primary in the breast show the same predilection for nerve infiltration so familiar in adenoid cystic carcinomas of salivary glands.

In contrast to experience with this neoplasm in other parts of the body, metastasis to regional lymph nodes from adenoid cystic carcinoma of breast is extraordinarily rare. There have been only one or two documented instances of lymph node involvement and only one or two documented fatalities as a direct result of this neoplasm.

A group of these we studied some years ago were like other breast cancers clinically, but at the time of follow-up, all of these patients were living and well and none had evidence of axillary lymph node metastasis.

Being aware of the biologic behavior of this type of neoplasm might make possible more conservative forms of therapy. This is not really a practical problem, however, because the lesion is so rare. The 21 examples in our group were found in something over 5000 mammary cancers.

A more familiar favorable mammary carcinoma is mucinous carcinoma. Again, these are well-circumscribed lesions. Halsted was familiar with this carcinoma, and he reported that they have a sort of swishing feel on palpation. These are well-differentiated neoplasms with the epithelial component swimming, floating, or suspended in a sea of mucin.

This type of mammary cancer is most often found in older women in this country. In Japan, they are much more frequent and occur in a younger age group. One explanation for the favorable prognosis of mammary cancer in Japan may be that they have a higher percentage of favorable types of carcinoma.

There can be admixture of other types of mammary cancers with mucinous carcinoma. We studied a group that, so far as we could tell, were all pure and without admixture. Only six of these patients died of tumor and two of them had second primaries in opposite breasts that were typical infiltrating duct cancers. In three, we did not really have adequate histologic material to evaluate. One had only one section from a tumor 10 cm in diameter. Thus, of the six patients who died, only one can be said with assurance to have had a pure mucinous carcinoma, emphasizing that these are favorable tumors.

Medullary carcinoma of the breast is probably the commonest of the mammary cancers that have significantly more favorable prognoses. This type, too, shows geographic differences. In studies from England, there is about twice the incidence of medullary carcinoma as in series from this country.

Grossly, these are again well-circumscribed tumors. Frequently there are large areas of necrosis centrally, and they can be confused with abscesses or fat necrosis. A dense lymphocytic infiltrate separates the lighter, larger neoplastic cells. The cells often show strange mitotic figures and have terrible looking nuclei, but nevertheless, these tumors have a favorable prognosis. Whether the prognosis is as good in 10 years as it appears in 5 has been questioned, but most series suggest that they are, in fact very favorable.

Another breast cancer which has a favorable prognosis is what we call, with dramatic lack of imagination, well-differentiated carcinoma. Others call them tubular cancers, but serial sections show that the typical structures are not tubules but glands. Another synonym for this lesion is "orderly carcinoma." In a group we reviewed, the average size was smaller than that of most breast cancers (it was just under 2 cm). The incidence of axillary metastasis in this group was 30%, but in only two instances was more than one lymph node involved. Only one patient is known to have died of her cancer. Another was living with tumor, but was lost to follow-up. Even if we presume her dead, that is only 2 of 33 patients in this category who died of mammary cancer.

It is a little difficult to discuss the prognosis of papillary carcinoma. When it becomes invasive, it looks just like ordinary duct carcinoma; if it is not invasive, obviously the prognosis is favorable. It is hard to know exactly what is being evaluated by survival figures in papillary cancer. Most papillary carcinomas have a favorable prognosis, either because they are frequently noninvasive at the time of discovery or because their inherent biologic behavior is relatively indolent.

I would like to conclude with a plea that comparative survival studies of breast cancer recognize that there are different kinds of breast cancer that have different natural histories and take this factor into consideration when comparing results.

Mammography and the Symptomatic Breast: A Panel Discussion

Moderator: JAMES T. DeLUCA, M.D.
CHARLES W. HAYDEN, M.D.
HENRY P. LEIS, Jr., M.D.
DAVID D. PAULUS, M.D.
GEORGE P. ROSEMOND, M.D.

DR. DE LUCA: Our panel is assembled and ready to answer questions from the audience.

QUESTION: I have two questions for Dr. Paulus. One is how long after you inject the contrast medium do you have to get your study done? The second question is how well can you distinguish malignancy from intraductal papilloma?

DR. PAULUS: I shall answer the second question first. The chances are that I cannot differentiate between intraductal papilloma and a carcinoma in a small intraductal duct lesion by contrast injection. In answer to the first question, you have 5 or 10 minutes after injection in which you can get good detail. After 15 or 20 minutes, absorption and discharge result in loss of the contrast medium.

QUESTION: If you cannot predict too well whether a lesion is malignant or benign, you are only helping the surgeon in localizing the lesion. Is that really worth it to him?

DR. PAULUS: One advantage is showing the exact distribution of that duct system as well as the localization of an abnormality, or tumor, or filling defect. Once a tumor gets to be a centimeter in size, it is usually fairly evident on the plain images. Contrast mammography is most useful in detecting 1 to

79

3 mm lesions within a duct. At that stage, all I can tell is that there is a tumor there. The chances, of course, are that it is benign. The study shows how big the lesion is and how to approach it surgically.

QUESTION: If the contrast mammogram just shows duct ectasia, can the patient be spared an exploration?

DR. LEIS: Duct ectasias are so characteristic on clinical examination that we have not felt it necessary to do contrast mammography to confirm this diagnosis. These cases respond to conservative medical therapy, and we have not resorted to contrast mammography when the diagnosis of duct ectasia is obvious. Contrast mammography is most useful in younger patients with serous, sanguineous, or bloody nipple discharge. In such patients it is preferable, if possible, to remove only the involved duct and a wedge of adjacent breast tissue. We like to know exactly where the lesion is and how far down it goes. In patients past the childbearing age, I prefer to do a complete central duct excision.

QUESTION: Did I understand you to say that every patient with either bloody, serous, or sanguineous discharge, surgical intervention is called for?

DR. LEIS: In general, except for women in the childbearing age, if the patient has a spontaneous serous, sanguineous, bloody, or watery discharge, I advise central duct exploration, regardless of the mammogram, regardless of the cytology, and regardless of whether I can feel a lump. This does not, of course, apply to a patient in the last trimester of pregnancy when a discharge of this type would probably be due to engorgement. Such patients need only be carefully followed.

QUESTION: Dr. Paulus, would you discuss the contraindications to contrast mammography?

DR. PAULUS: I do not know that there are any definite contraindications. I have never had any complications.

DR. JEROME URBAN: There is one point that has not been sufficiently stressed, and that is that all these intraductal lesions are multicentric. I do not understand the point of doing segmental resection. If you are going to remove a duct you should take the whole duct system. We have done this routinely since 1947 and have not had any trouble with young women. If they become pregnant, the breast dries up quickly. It is important to have good hemostasis so you can follow the involved ducts out to the periphery of involvement. I prefer to use a radial incision. The closure is better when a large section of tissue has been removed.

DR. ROSEMOND: We also use the radial incision. In young women, however, we prefer just to do excision of the involved duct. We consider spontaneous discharge somewhat in the same category as a dominant mass, and we explore the pertinent area. I can recall only two patients I have had to reexplore because the discharge was not stopped.

DR. LEIS: I want to emphasize what Dr. Urban has said. We have found, even in our intraductal papillomas, a multiplicity rate of over 14%. Fibrocystic disease of the papillomatous type is extemely multicentric, including all of the duct areas. This is why we prefer to do a complete central duct excision.

QUESTION: We have heard about joint management and combined studies of breast cancer patients. How is this to be accomplished in the usual practice situation? Who is going to set the guidelines for seeing patients in some definite kind of management program?

DR. DE LUCA: What you are asking is a multiphasic question to which nobody has the answer. The team approach is a necessity, as has been recognized for the last decade. It is essential that each discipline contribute its expertise with full cooperation if patient care is to be optimal. This is especially true in the patient who has only the roentgen findings of breast cancer without any clinical manifestations. In most communities, it is the surgeon who has the initiative and the ultimate responsibility in such a situation. He, after all, must remove the area in question for microscopic analysis. It is the radiologist who contributes, following biopsy, specimen radiography to aid in the detection of these early cancers.

I do not know whether I have answered your question completely, but time has now run out and we must adjourn.

PART THREE:

DETECTING ASYMPTOMATIC BREAST CANCER

Present Potential
and Ultimate Objectives
of Screening Programs

WILLIAM M. MARKEL, M.D.

In February 1972 the Board of Directors of the American Cancer Society, after a report from its Breast Cancer Task Force, approved the concept of a major program of earlier breast cancer detection. It was planned to establish 12 demonstration projects, 3 in each of the four ACS areas, and to spend $1 million a year to accomplish this. Each of these projects was to examine 5000 women a year for two years. The goal was to discover breast cancer in asymptomatic women when the disease is most amenable to treatment, and thereby to change the mortality that has lived with us for so many years. It was recognized that this had to be more than just a medical project. There had to be an associated public education campaign, a professional education campaign, and a public information campaign: public education to reinforce the concept of periodic health examinations, professional education to help physicians understand the value of mammography and thermography, and public information to bring in the screenees.

The working assumptions on which this plan was based were (a) that earlier detection and prompt and adequate treatment lead to improved patient survival, and (b) that the combination of history, clinical, radiographic, and thermographic examination is the most effective program for earlier detection now available.

The major objective was to demonstrate the feasibility and the practicability of repeated screening for the early detection of breast cancer. Another objective was to identify target populations for future efforts on the basis of risk factors. A third objective was to evaluate the variations in techniques required by variations in demographic characteristics, socioeconomic status, accessibility to medical care, and health attitudes in order to gain patient acceptance and participation. Finally, we hoped to explore and demonstrate, wherever possible, the role of allied health professionals in screening.

In the summer and fall of 1972, the National Cancer Institute became interested in the proposed program, and we began to work on a cooperative program, expanding the project from the original 12 centers to 20. The NCI helped to develop a site visiting system and cooperated with the City Science Development Group in Philadelphia to standardize records and data retrieval.

Approximately 75 institutions responded to the initial request for applications. Some 20 of these were excluded from further consideration, after site visits by area medical vice-presidents of the ACS demonstrated obvious deficiencies. Fifty-four of the centers were site visited by teams that included ACS volunteers and 20 were approved. Recently, an additional 7 have been funded.

Of the 27, 11 are now in operation. Nine more have negotiated contracts, and 7 more will have their contracts written within the next several months. All 27 will be operative by summer or fall of this year.

The evaluation of each of these applicants depended heavily on the kind of follow-up procedures they were willing to establish. There is not much point to detecting something if you cannot also arrange for adequate treatment. A numerical system was used in evaluation and roughly one-third of the credit had to do with the professional aspects of the applicant's facility, such as their experience in doing mammography, thermography, and breast examination. Another one-third of the points had to do with the organizational support. Did the administration of the facility function effectively? Would they provide space? Had they experience in screening programs? Did they know their community? The final one-third of the credit had to do with the relationship between facility and the local ACS division. Were volunteers from the ACS familiar with the hospital? Had they had joint programs previously? Was ACS prepared to do the transportation and to help to get women in?

When all of the projects are in operation, just under 300,000 women will be entered into the system. Each of these women will be examined annually (or more often if there is a special circumstance) for five years, and then each will be followed, without examination, for another five years.

One important question, not strictly medical, is how do you get different population groups to come in? When we launch a program in New York City, *The New York Times* reports it well, and the people who read *The Times* come in to the project. They are not necessarily, however, the people we want. They usually have their own doctors, are usually medically oriented, and are under medical surveillance. One of the chores for the ACS is to find ways to motivate a broader segment of the population, not just middle and upper-class people who are already motivated.

We have included in each project a breast self-examination objective. Originally it was planned to show films on breast self-examination and to give lectures. Then came the Gallup report and we discovered that films and literature do not persuade women to examine their breasts. A physician has to instruct them. So, we have to revise our plans and find new ways to get breast self-examination taught and implemented at these projects.

Another unanswered question is whether the allied health professionals necessary to carry the load will be accepted by patients. Early reports certainly indicate that they will. In some of the projects, they were not accepted because the medical community did not want allied health professions in this field. I am not promoting them, but if we are going to make these projects practical and feasible, it is going to be necessary to use paramedical personnel. Perhaps we will have to learn something about professional education techniques.

We have been somewhat staggered by the public response to date. As soon as the first story about a screening facility hit the headlines, the facility was swamped for appointments and booked six months in advance. This is an unhealthy situation. It is obviously undesirable to build a fire under people and then have to say, "We would like to serve you but you'll have to wait for six months." This is an unsolved problem.

A similar problem has to do with the hardware. It needs to be evaluated from the professional standpoint, of course. But it also needs to be evaluated logistically. How much down time is there? How fast does the manufacturer send a representative out to fix the machine? This is important because when there are appointments scheduled for weeks ahead and equipment is inoperative for three days, the appointments have to be juggled.

We are a long way away from analysis of our data and from being sure that our data are correct, but we already have some early figures that seem to indicate some trends. The Virginia Mason Clinic Project, for example, has done 2500 women from September 1973 through February 1974. They are moving at better than 20 examinations per day, the number needed to achieve 5000 per year. In those 2500 women they found 16 cancers, a little more than anticipated, but of those, 5 were occult. Of the 16, 11 had negative nodes. Thus it appears that we are finding some cancers earlier than they would have been found by physical examination alone, and earlier than the woman would have found them herself. These are early figures, and this is the way the trend seems to be going.

At the same time, we are facing some problems. We are not, as alluded to previously, getting the total population we desire. Some women are coming because their own doctors are doing film mammograms and they want to have xeromammograms. Or, a symptomatic woman wants to check on her physician when he says, "You have a mass and you should have a biopsy because it is indicated." Young women want to have mammography done and feel slighted when they are processed through without mammography. The medical history forms inherited from the NCI are overwhelming in detail, and in the time it requires to execute them. The projects, however, are evolving and we are facing these problems on a daily basis.

There is need constantly to review our long-range goals. Will we be able to identify high risk groups on the basis of data obtained from these projects? We cannot expect to be able to screen 50 million women in our lifetimes with the procedures now available. Above all, we must now zero in on some kind of high risk identification. Real economies will be necessary if there is to be an acceptable cost-benefit ratio. It is easy to say that one cancer detected is worth all the money in the world, but, practically speaking, unless costs can be reduced within reason, third parties will not pay, insurance companies will not pay, and we are going to be in trouble.

Can we interest industry? Can we convince industry that the medical profession thinks this is the way to go? Can we find a role for mammographic screeners? Can we determine the optimal frequency for screening? Are some tests going to be better for certain types of bodies and certain ages than others? Obviously, we are not going to be able to screen the whole country with our 27 centers. Will the existence of these 27 demonstration projects make other people want to do likewise? All of these are questions to which we need answers.

Still another question concerns the expertise of the people who are suddenly doing all this mammography. When something balloons and snowballs quickly, there are always those who become involved without being properly trained or completely briefed. We are concerned and thus are setting up training and review programs for the project directors and their associates, as well as quality control measures.

We have financial problems. We have professional problems. We are living with day-by-day logistic problems. But hopefully, a major step has been taken toward changing the breast cancer mortality rate that we have lived with for many years.

The Histopathology of Clinically Occult Mammary Carcinoma

PAUL PETER ROSEN, M.D.

I t is almost as difficult to decide what an occult breast cancer is as it is to settle on a definition of "early breast cancer." There is a tendency to adopt easy-to-use phrases such as these, but they lack specific definitions and are open to varied interpretations.

The term early breast cancer is used to designate lesions confined to the breast, small cancers of undefined size, or some combination of the two. Whatever an early breast cancer is, it is not necessarily occult. Cancers confined to the breast tend to be smaller than those with metastases, but many are palpable masses. The terms early and occult are, therefore, not necessarily interchangeable.

It has been said that an occult lesion is one that was missed by the previous observer. Obviously, what one calls occult cancer depends on the selectivity and sensitivity of the method of detection. If a patient is unaware of a lesion that is palpable to an examining physician, is it occult? What about a lesion that is visible in a mammogram but not evident to patient or examining physician? Or a palpable lesion that cannot be identified in a mammogram?

In the future, the concept of occult carcinoma may be extended even further. New techniques, probably based on immunology, could provide forewarning that breast cancer is likely to develop in a given individual even before it can be recognized by current histological criteria. Some of the epithelial proliferations that are not recognized as cancer today may then be considered to be occult neoplasia. Future studies of the relationship between epithelial proliferations and occult cancer will require not only retrospective clinicopathologic analyses but also the development of entirely new noninvasive techniques that have the reliability, ease of performance, and lack of complications of the cervical Pap smear. No procedure now in use fulfills these requirements, largely because of the relatively inaccessible and dispersed nature of the mammary epithelium.

With these limitations in mind, it is possible to suggest a working definition of occult breast cancer and to describe the types of lesions encountered in that context.

The majority of breast carcinomas are found by patients because they feel a lump. The presence of a mass is often the only symptom. If an occult breast cancer is one that is asymptomatic, then a minimal definition requires that the lesion not be apparent to the patient. This can be refined somewhat to the concept of *clinically* occult cancer, which is definable as one not detected either by the patient or on physical examination.

Until the development of effective radiographic techniques, clinically occult breast cancers were unexpected histologic findings in biopsies performed for lesions which themselves proved to be benign. A substantial number of such cancers can now be visualized by mammography.

Many, but definitely not all, clinically occult breast carcinomas are noninvasive. By definition, in situ or noninvasive carcinoma appears by light microscopy to be confined to the epithelium from which it originated in the duct, lobule, or both.

Clinically occult invasive carcinomas are usually ductal in origin. There are rare instances in which infiltrating lobular carcinoma can produce diffuse disease in the breast and remain asymptomatic because there is no discrete mass. Except for occasional examples of the special well-differentiated type described as tubular carcinoma, clinically occult infiltrating duct lesions have no unusual histologic features other than their small size. It is uncommon for any of the other specialized histologic types of cancer to present as clinically occult lesions. Perhaps this is because they are infrequent to begin with.

A substantial number of clinically occult cancers detected by mammography contain calcifications. Recently, Rogers and Powell reported their results in 72 patients who had clinically normal breasts and abnormal mammograms. Most of the occult cancers they found were ductal in origin. Radiologically, 83.5% of the cancers contained calcifications, and in 63.5% of the cases calcifications were the only abnormal radiologic finding.

Calcifications are only one of many radiologic signs of breast cancer, and, in fact, the majority of calcifications seen in mammograms are associated with benign lesions. Calcifications, however, provide a convenient marker for tracing occult lesions. In a substantial number of cases, they are the only evidence of disease. Through the use of specimen radiography, calcifications can serve as a means of identifying and localizing cancers that are not palpable in the pathology laboratory.

Specimen radiography is not a new procedure. Its use has been described by Egan and others over the years ever since mammography became available. Some years ago Dr. Ruth Snyder and I reported our experience with specimen radiography of biopsy specimens that had been diagnosed as benign after routine gross and microscopic examination. By studying radiographs of the original intact specimens, Dr. Snyder was able to pinpoint areas with microcalcifications. In about one-half of the cases, the areas with calcifications had been included in sections already taken. In the other cases, radiographs of the residual tissue allowed us to localize the areas in question. Histological study of these foci revealed 27 carcinomas. The majority of these were ductal, usually intraductal lesions with central necrosis, so-called comedocarcinomas. By contrast, the calcifications that led us to lobular lesions usually were present in contiguous cysts or sclerosing adenosis. This may simply represent a fortuitous association.

We have continued to do routine specimen radiography since reporting our results in 1971, but the yield has been greatly reduced. This can be attributed to several changes that have occurred. First, the majority of patients now have preoperative mammograms. Second, there have been substantial technical improvements in the quality of mammography in the last five years, so that clinical films have nearly the same clarity as specimen radiographs. Third, specimen radiographs are always obtained during surgery if a biopsy is done for a clinically occult lesion detected by mammography. Preoperative mammography combined with specimen radiography during surgery in selected cases can now detect most cancers that had previously been found by routine specimen radiography. If clinical mammography has not been performed, routine specimen radiography is still a useful procedure in certain cases, such as contralateral biopsies of patients with proven cancer in one breast.

Between June 1971 and August 1973 we studied 125 consecutive breast biopsies performed in cases where a lesion with calcifications was seen in the mammogram and was interpreted as suggestive of carcinoma and there was no corresponding palpable tumor. The same histological types of carcinoma were found in this material as have turned up as occult lesions in prior studies, namely, noninvasive carcinoma of ducts and lobules and minimally invasive duct carcinomas. Overall, there were 32 carcinomas, representing 25% of the 125 biopsies.

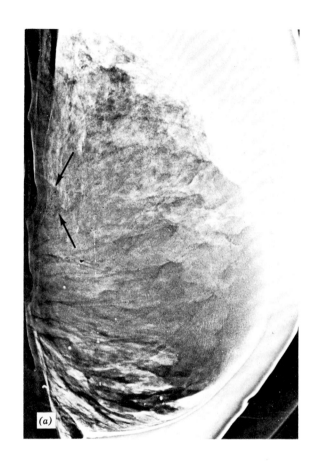

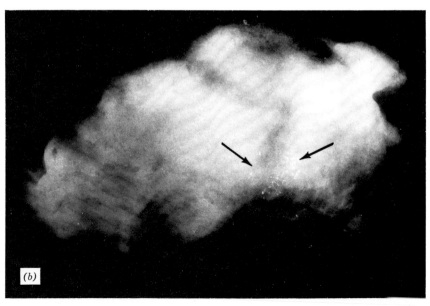

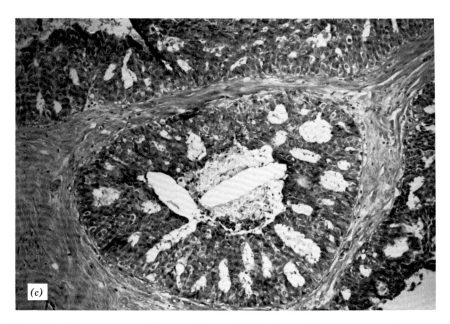

Figure 1. This case exemplifies one form of clinically occult mammary carcinoma. *(a)* Xeroradiogram obtained as part of annual examination of an elderly woman revealed a group of punctate calcifications (between arrows) deep within the breast. No mass was palpable. *(b)* Radiograph of specimen obtained at surgery shows the corresponding area with calcifications that proved to be *(c)* an intraductal carcinoma.

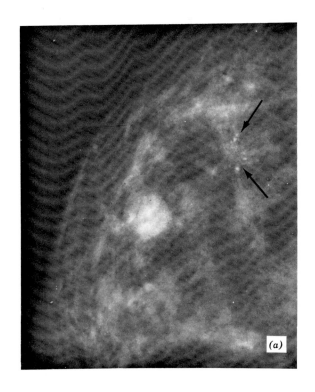

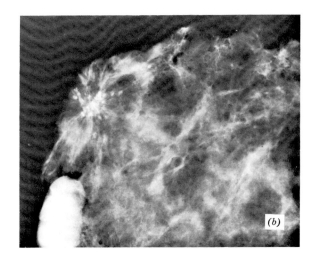

94

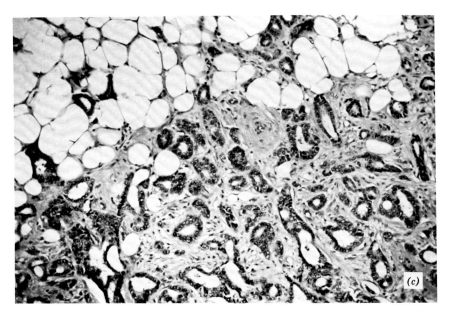

Figure 2. Another form of clinically occult carcinoma is seen in this patient who felt a small mass in her breast. This nodule was visualized in a mammogram *(a)* which also revealed a nonpalpable small stellate area that contained calcifications deeper in the breast (single arrow). Both lesions can be seen in the specimen radiograph *(b)*. The larger tumor was a fibroadenoma while the clinically occult lesion *(c)* was an infiltrating duct carcinoma.

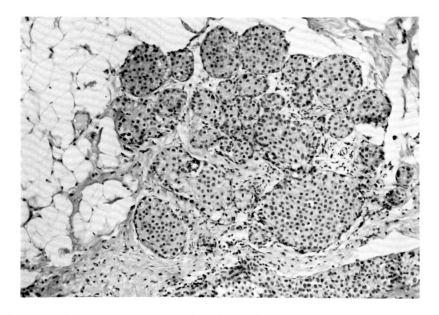

Figure 3. Lobular carcinoma in situ is a form of clinically occult carcinoma that is usually found unexpectedly at the time of histologic examination.

Effect of Screening on Survivals

LOUIS VENET, M.D.
SAM SHAPIRO
PHILIP STRAX, M.D.
WANDA VENET, R.N.

The study described in this paper was begun in December 1963 at the Health Insurance Plan of Greater New York with the objective of determining whether periodic screening for breast cancer by means of mammography and clinical examination would result in a reduction in mortality from this disease. In our early papers, we described in detail the methodology and reported on detection rates of breast cancer found by screening. Subsequent reports recorded the histology, rates of nodal involvement, sizes of lesions, and the rates of breast cancer detection as the annual screenings progressed. At the First National Breast Cancer Conference, we described the relative effectiveness of clinical and mammographic examination in detecting breast cancer. ·We concluded then that "clinical examination and x-ray mammography contribute independently to the detection of breast cancer and neither one can be dispensed with in the search for early disease." Preliminary mortality data suggesting a reduction in the death rate as a result of screening were presented in 1971 at the Second National Breast Cancer Conference. In 1972 at the Seventh National Cancer Conference, the observations covering a follow-up period of five years reinforced the conclusions of the earlier reports that women in the

From the Department of Research and Statistics, Health Insurance Plan of Greater New York (HIP). Supported in part by the U.S. Public Health Service under contracts PH43-63-49 and NIH 69-88.

screening program have a substantially lower mortality than a similarly constituted control group. At present, after an additional year of observation, the conclusion remains the same: screening results in a reduction in mortality of approximately one-third in the study group as compared with the control group.

The methodology of the study has involved the random selection of two samples, each consisting of approximately 31,000 women aged 40–64, from the HIP population. The 31,000 women of the study group were asked to appear for screening examinations; the control women were not. Of the study group, 20,166 responded initially and were invited to return at annual intervals for three additional screening examinations (unless earlier follow-up was recommended). All examinations have been completed.

These examinations were conducted at 23 medical group centers throughout the greater New York area. The physical examinations were performed, for the most part, by group surgeons. A modified Egan technique was used for obtaining mammograms, and this has yielded a high degree of reproductibility. The clinicians and radiologists recorded their findings and recommendations independently, each without knowledge of the other's observations. Women in the control group followed the usual practices in receiving medical care.

As stated, about 21,000 women, or 65% of the study group, responded and participated in the initial screening examinations. Of these women, 80% appeared for their first annual reexamination, 74% for the second annual reexamination, and 69% for a third annual reexamination. Only 12% of the women failed to return for any of the annual reexaminations. Sixty percent participated in all four examinations, (the initial plus three annual rescreenings), and 28% had two or three examinations. The entire population (study women who were screened, as well as those who refused screening, and the control women) has been followed for at least five years following entry into the study. In these five years, 299 breast cancers have been diagnosed among the 31,000 study women (225 in the screened group and 74 in the group who refused screenings), and 285 breast cancers have been diagnosed among the controls. The rates at which breast cancer has been detected and confirmed histologically are presented in Table 1.

As a result of screening, 132 breast cancers were detected and confirmed—44 on radiologic evidence alone, 59 on clinical evidence alone, and 29 on independent recommendations from both clinician and radiologist. Table 2 depicts the situation that would have occurred had either modality been omitted from the screening program. Forty-five percent of the cancers would have been missed had the clinical examination been omitted, 33% with the omission of mammography. Furthermore, the two modalities were unequal in their ability to detect breast cancer in women under 50. The clinical examination in this group proved to be more effec-

Table 1   Breast Cancer Detection Rates Five Years of Observation from Date of Entry

	Breast Cancers	
Population	Number	Rate per 1000[a]
Study (screened)	225	2.34
Detection due to initial examination[b]	55	2.73
Detection due to annual reexamination	77	1.49
Detection not due to screening[c]	93	0.92
Study (refused screening)	74	1.45
Control	285	1.87

[a] Rate of detection due to initial screening is per 1000 women examined; other rates are per 1000 person-years.

[b] A total of 20,166 women had initial screening examinations.

[c] Includes only cases diagnosed in the course of regular medical care; case detection not due to follow-up of screening findings. Also included are four cases confirmed on biopsy among women with positive screening results who refused surgery for more than one year.

Table 2   Effect of Omitting a Screening Modality by Age Group

	Percentage of Breast Cancers in Age Group Missed	
Age at Diagnosis	If Omit Clinical	If Omit Mammography
TOTAL	45	33
40—49	61	19
50—59	40	42
60+	39	31

tive. In women over 50, on the other hand, the two modalities were similar.

Of particular interest are the results of clinical reexamination of patients considered negative by screening physician examination but for whom biopsy was recommended upon an independent reading of the mammograms. There were 44 such cases, and of these, the biopsy recommendation was based on the presence of a mass in 28 and the presence of microcalcifications in 16. When these patients were reexamined with the radiologic reports and films available, in only 3 of the 16 cases with calcifications was a palpable mass recorded. However, a clinical mass was found in 19 of the 28 patients with radiologic masses (Table 3). It is a fact that under screening conditions, clinicians may fail to detect some breast cancers that are apparent radiologically. Conversely, as we have reported previously, under screening conditions, cancers may be detected by clinicians even though there is no evidence of malignancy on the mammograms. Reexamination of the films following biopsy proof that cancer is present in such instance produces no change in interpretation.

Table 3 Results of Clinical Reexamination in 44 Breast Cancers Detected Radiologically[a]

Clinical Reexamination	X-ray Screening Findings		
	Total	Mass	Calcifications
Total	44	28	16
Negative	9	3	6
Indefinite	13	6	7
Mass	22	19	3

[a] Initial screening evidence for biopsy was radiologic finding of mass or calcifications.

An extensive follow-up program enables us to determine the rate of breast cancer diagnosis in the study group between screening examinations and subsequent to the final screening. Table 4 indicates the breast cancers found within 12 months after screening and those at subsequent intervals. Of the 93 cases, 45 occurred within a year of screening and an additional 48 between 12 and 59 months later. Of the 45 detected less than 12 months after screening, 35, or 78%, were diagnosed between 6 and 11 months.

Table 4 Breast Cancers[a] Found Within 12 Months After Screening (Not Result of Screening Group)

Interval Post Screening (months)	Number	Percentage
Total	45	100
< 2	0	0
2—3	7	16
4—5	3	7
6—11	35	78

[a] A total of 48 additional cases detected 12 to 59 months after screening examination.

Deaths are identified through intensive follow-up of confirmed breast cancer cases, and by matching death records on file in various health departments (New York City, upstate New York, New Jersey, Connecticut, and Florida) against the total file of study women, including those who have failed to have a screening reexamination, and the file of control women. As a final check in the process, several months after the fifth anniversary of each woman's entry date, an attempt has been made through a mail survey to determine whether the woman has breast cancer not previously known to the study staff.

Since the study and control groups are random selections of equal size from the Health Insurance Plan members, comparisons involving numbers of deaths during the defined periods provide the same information as rates. At present, with six years of follow-up after the date of entry of each patient into the study, there have been 56 deaths attributable to breast cancer in the study group and 88 in the control group. The deaths in the study group include those occurring among patients who were screened and those not screened combined. The difference between this figure and the number of deaths in the control group is statistically significant (Figure 1).

Another approach to measuring mortality experience involves the use of the case fatality rate, which is the mortality from all causes among women with histologically confirmed breast cancer. The case fatality rates have been calculated allowing for one year's lead time gained in breast cancer detection as a result of screening. That is, a five year case fatality rate for the study group is a composite of a six year mortality among all other cases in the study. Figure 2 reveals that the fatality rate in the study group is 28% as compared with 42% in the control group. Again, in these comparisons, the

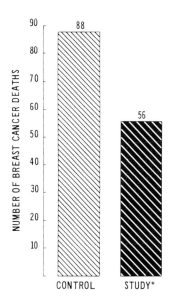

*Includes deaths among women screened and
those who refused screening.

Figure 1. Deaths due to breast cancer, six years of follow-up after entry to study.

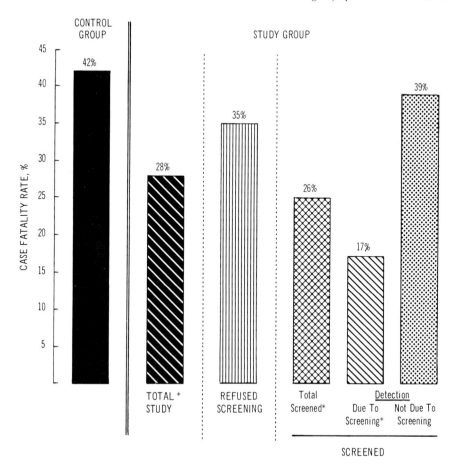

*Allowance made for 1 year lead time in cancer detection due to screening.

Figure 2. Five year case fatality rates among breast cancer cases.

study group includes both screened and not screened women. Considering only those cases detected through screening, the case fatality rate becomes much lower—17%. Among the 44 cases detected by mammographic evidence only, there has been only one death in the period of follow-up for this report. Deaths due to causes other than breast cancer (Table 5) are remarkably similar in all categories in both the study and control groups.

When we first reported the five year results showing a reduction in mortality in the study group, we predicted that the development of practical programs to screen for breast cancer would assume a high priority. In addition, we stated that ". . . further research that would lead to more efficient screening modalities, increased use of paramedical personnel, and identification of women at high risk for breast cancer" would also receive

Table 5   Death Rate by Cause of Death (Excluding Breast Cancer) Five Year Follow-up After Entry (Rate per 10,000 Person-years)

Cause of Death	Control	Study
All causes (excluding breast cancer)	54.3	53.9
Malignant neoplasms	17.3	16.2
Digestive system	6.3	6.0
Genitourinary system	4.9	3.9
Other	6.1	6.3
Circulatory system	24.9	24.0
Other	12.1	13.7

NOTE. Data refer to mortality over a five-year period among women with entry dates through December 31, 1965, representing 82% of the total population in study and control groups.

increasing attention. Recently, the National Cancer Institute and the American Cancer Society have joined forces to subsidize 27 breast cancer demonstration units throughout the United States. Our own group is continuing the intensive follow-up of the patients in the study and control groups to determine whether the mortality differences observed will persist after long follow-up. In addition, under a contract with the National Cancer Institute, we are now attempting to evaluate the role of thermography in screening for breast cancer. It is too early to report on this project, other than to state that two screening centers have already been established as part of the program, one at Beth Israel Medical Center (to screen HIP patients in the Bronx and Manhattan) and other at the LaGuardia Hospital in Queens (to screen patients in that borough and in Nassau County). We hope to report results of this research at subsequent meetings.

Modalities, Methods, and Management for Screening Programs

PHILIP STRAX, M.D.

Mass screening of apparently well women for breast cancer differs in approach, methodology, and results from examination of symptomatic women. As physicians, we have been trained to diagnose and treat disease. Medical school curricula pay little more than lip service to preventive medicine. The average clinician soothes his conscience by approving preventive measures in principle, but ignoring them in practice. We are all so busy caring for the sick that we have little time or interest in preventing illness or finding it when unsuspected by the patient. This is particularly true of measures for the control of cancer. Mass screening for earlier detection of breast cancer has come to the fore because of the one-third reduction in mortality produced in a six year follow-up. In that program, 88 women died in the control group and only 56 in the study group when randomly selected women aged 40 to 64 received an initial and three annual examinations that included palpation and mammography.

To reduce mortality in a deadly disease is certainly a desired result, but our attitude towards screening sometimes defeats our purpose. Our training and expertise make us ready to give time freely to the differential diagnosis of a symptomatic patient, but examining endless numbers of normal women we find boring and time consuming. Looking for needles in haystacks is to be relegated to lesser mortals or to machines. We thus turn to paramedical persons or to devices for help.

The cost factor must also be introduced. Is the gain worth the expense? Should a screening program for breast cancer have priority over other health programs? Is the cost of finding an unsuspected breast cancer or even of saving a life from breast cancer by screening too great to make it worthwhile? In symptomatic women such problems as radiation dosage, duration of examination, or proportion of benign to malignant results at operation are of little importance, but they loom large in the screening process.

Let us approach the problem by asking and answering some questions commonly brought up.

Why should we screen for breast cancer?

Some day the basic cause of breast cancer will be found and either a specific preventive will be developed or we may find the magic bullet to destroy the cancer cell wherever it may be. When either goal is achieved, the problem of breast cancer will be solved. Today, unfortunately, we have only a death rate which has been stationary for 40 years, and the data from the study conducted by the Health Insurance Plan of Greater New York (HIP) is the only light in the tunnel. Mass screening for breast cancer is the only practical means available for finding cancer at a time when present treatment methods are curative and can lower mortality. That is why we must do mass screening for breast cancer. It is the only hope available to save the lives of more women with this disease.

What is screening?

Screening is simply a procedure to detect undiagnosed, unsuspected disease. The screener may be the patient, a physician, an allied health professional, or a machine. The screenee is any individual who may have the disease sought. The screening process may include one or more modalities. Screening does not result in a definitive diagnosis. That is the domain of the physician. Thus breast cancer screening is only screening for abnormalities. The physician, not the screening process, evaluates the abnormalities and makes the differentiation between benign and malignant disease.

At present, the patient herself is the screener 90 to 95% of the time. She detects her disease because of a lump, pain, or discharge, and brings the condition to the attention of a physician. For this reason, breast self-examination is and will remain a vital modality in breast cancer screening. The clinician makes a differential diagnosis and proceeds to treatment. Occasionally a physician may be the screener when, for example, he finds a lesion unsuspected by the patient during a routine examination or in a breast opposite to one with symptoms.

By definition, the detection process involves many individuals who have no disease. It should, therefore, be quick, readily available, economical, acceptable to the screenee, and harmless. It must also find the disease early enough in order that it can be more easily and effectively treated.

In breast cancer, earlier detection has been proved by the HIP study to lead to lowered mortality. It therefore behooves us to use clinical examination, mammography, and thermography in breast cancer screening and, if possible, add other modalities when they show promise. Detection of earlier lesions usually brings increased difficulty in detection. The more and the finer the sieves, the more patients with disease will be detected. New modalities provide additional sieves, and should be added to the screening process as soon as their usefulness is demonstrated, provided that the added modality does not adversely affect time, effort, expense, risk, patient acceptance, and does not lead to an inordinate number of false positives and unnecessary surgical procedures.

Whom do we screen for breast cancer?

Only 7 of every 100 females will develop breast cancer in their lifetimes. If we knew who they were, the screening process would be simplified. Factors indicating high risk are being sought, but there is still no one factor nor even a practical combination of factors that help. Factors indicating a risk of twice or three times average spread over the lifetime of a woman are tantalizing indicators, but are hardly of practical significance. The sad truth is that in the light of present meager knowledge, all women in the United States are at risk after the age of 30 and that the risk increases with age. It is hoped that markers may be found in such things as urinary or blood hormone ratios that will delineate true high risk groups. In the meantime screening for breast cancer is a need and a right of all women over 35 or 40. Screening is also an educational process. Younger women respond enthusiastically to the call for breast screening. Such women should not be turned away, but should be examined and encouraged to continue examinations.

How frequently should women be screened for breast cancer?

The answer to this still eludes us. Most investigators believe at present that once a year is practical, and that special provision should be made for those obviously at greater risk, such as women with previous mastectomies or markedly positive family histories. Should a positive thermogram be the sole positive finding, this also calls for more frequent examinations. Provision must also be made for the input of the clinician, who may be concerned with breasts of special consistency or texture. At present, there are no definite data that indicate how frequently screening should be done.

Where should we screen?

The answer is obvious: wherever the women at risk happen to be. Screening should be conducted in a place appropriate to the women being examined.

Most middle and upper income women have established relationships with medical institutions. For low income groups, a hospital setting may be anathema. Such women should be examined in housing projects or churches or community rooms on a mobile basis. We must make the screening process available and accessible to those we seek. We are delivering a public health service and the screenees are our guests, not the recipients of handouts.

How is breast cancer screening done? What modalities should be used?

The demonstration that screening can reduce mortality led to the foundation of the Guttman Institute in 1968. Its objective is the development of more practical, more efficient, and more economical methods of screening. Studies of improved mammographic techniques using the Senograph with a molybdenum anode tube and of thermography have produced a practical screening technique. This takes about 20 minutes, costs about $20 per woman (when 10,000 to 15,000 women are screened per year), and includes the following:

1. An interview for demographic, menstrual, family, medication, and breast history. These data may lead to better understanding of high risk markers. Volunteers may be used to conduct and record the interviews.
2. Clinical examination done in the sitting and in the supine position by a physician or a trained paramedic. Allied health professionals are eminently suitable for the job. At the Guttman Institute, a physician is always present to supervise. Indoctrination of the woman in breast self-examination on a one-to-one basis is essential. It is done at this time by the physician or by the paramedic.
3. Mammography, done with the Senograph in the craniocaudad and mediolateral positions. About 10 women can be x-rayed per hour. Since it is anticipated that examinations will be repeated and since many of the screenees are in the younger age group, the dose of radiation accumulating in the breasts becomes important. Previous work indicates that an accumulated dose of 90 rads may increase the incidence of breast cancer. Since such a total should be avoided, doses of under 3 rads to a breast on any one examination should be used, and even less in women of 40 or under. The trend to so-called low dose techniques, using vacuum cassettes and dosages of 1 to 2 rads, seems to be a step in the right direction.
4. Thermography. This is particularly useful in the woman whose other findings are doubtful. It may also be a potential marker of high risk. It is especially appealing to women as a procedure and increases motivation to return. More data, such as will come from the HIP-Jefferson University study of thermography, are needed to put the procedure in proper perspective.

What results can be anticipated from screening?

Data from the Guttman Institute for 1971 and 1972 indicate that about 11 cancers per 1000 screenees were found on initial examinations. In subsequent examinations the figure dropped to 2 to 3 per 1000. Among cancers detected on initial screening, less than 50% were free of axillary node involvement, the usual situation in medical practice today. For those found by subsequent examination, the percentage was over 50% in 1971 and well over 60% in 1972. About 10% were "interval cancers," found within a year after a negative examination. Breast self-examination is essential to discover these lesions. Women who go through the Guttman Institute are alerted to the possibility of interval cancer and are urged to practice regular self-examination.

Currently about 2500 women per month are being examined at the Institute. A backlog of about a month is maintained. This is necessary to exclude the symptomatic woman who should be visiting her physician for prompt care.

How can women be persuaded to participate in screening?

A most important step in screening is motivation. The value of a detection method for breast cancer varies in proportion to its acceptance by women at risk. In screening, the anxiety created by a self found lump is lacking. Motivation of apparently well women to accept complete breast examination is not to be taken for granted. It needs to be developed, nurtured, and stimulated. Three important factors involved in motivation are

1. Awareness of the existence of the program.
2. Education to accept and even demand the program.
3. Availability and accessibility of the program.

The population at risk must be made aware of the existence of the detection program. Techniques used must match the type of women involved. Publicity via television and news media may be sufficient in English speaking areas, but in bilingual neighborhoods, multilingual flyers may prove more effective. In economically depressed regions, where women live with difficulty from day to day, medical attention is usually sought only for advanced conditions and preventive medicine is unknown. In such areas, personal contact, even a door-to-door campaign, may be needed. Contacts can also be made by community personnel or community churches. To make reluctant women aware of the screening facility and to carry out the educational process needed can tax the ingenuity of the agency involved.

Making women aware of a program must be accompanied by education to alert them to the need of the program in their lives. The examination must be made meaningful to the point that they will demand it, not just accept it. They must be so well indoctrinated before the initial examination and so well treated and informed at this first visit, that they will be eager for periodic study. The educational process must also involve talks to community groups, magazine articles, and even interviews by health aides on a one-to-one basis. It must include informational material given at the time of initial examination, explaining procedures and the value of the study, so that the screenee may carry the message to her friends.

The program must be easily and readily accessible to the women at risk. Transportation must be inexpensive or provided, if need be, by the facility. The facility must be large enough to meet the initial demand and have possibilities for expansion to meet increasing demands so that a reasonably small backlog can be maintained.

Screening centers are seldom located in low income areas or in institutions to which inner core people relate. Since this type of population resists medical care and especially preventive care, health fairs in such areas become all important.

The most extensive example of this type of screening is the outreach program of the Guttman Institute. Its main objective has been development of motivation of low income women to accept breast cancer screening. All outreach activities have an umbilical cord to the central facility, which is centrally located in Manhattan and convenient to all forms of transportation.

The outreach screening must be done with portable or transportable equipment. The four part examination is the same as that used at the central facility. The interview is performed by lay personnel, using forms similar to those at the central facility. Clinical examination is performed by clinicians recruited from neighboring medical institutions or by trained allied health personnel. Mammography is carried out using either a transportable 70 mm device, which can x-ray up to 20 women per hour with two views of each breast on economical 70 mm film with radiation dosage of 1 to 2 rads per exposure, or a transportable x-ray machine with a molybdenum anode tube, which operates on 110 volt current and produces acceptable mammograms on 8 x 10 film at radiation doses of 2 to 3 rads per exposure. A mobile van containing facilities for all four steps of the screening process is also used. The x-ray in this case is done by a Senograph with radiation doses of 2 to 3 rads per exposure using nonscreen film. This unit can process up to 70 women per day, is highly maneuverable, and is usually used close to a community center.

Thermography is done by an AGA Thermovision which is transportable and utilizes 70 mm film.

By using these devices in combination, up to 200 women have been screened with all modalities in one day. Provision is made for follow-up of suspicious cases through the central facility. The screenings are now being done on a periodic basis. Health fairs are held annually in the same communities. The response varies with the effort expended on education and with the economic level of the neighborhood. It is important to note that repeat screenings draw increased response.

Who Is the High Risk Patient?

E. CUYLER HAMMOND, Sc.D.

In a list of countries ranked by breast cancer death rates, the United States stands high but is not at the top. Some countries near the bottom of the list may be there because of lax reporting of mortality. There is, however, no doubt that breast cancer death rates are remarkably low in Japan. There has been much speculation as to the reason for this, but none of the suggested explanations have yet been confirmed by firm evidence.

A generation ago, cancer of the uterus was the leading cancer cause of death among American women. Today that distinction is held by breast cancer, and the change in relative status has been due almost entirely to a great decline in uterine cancer deaths. Needless to say, the aim of all of us is to bring about a similar decline in breast cancer mortality, which is nearly constant but seems to show some indication of rising.

Breast cancer death rates increase rapidly with age up to about 50. After that, the rise continues but much less rapidly. The rates are higher among white women in the United States than among black women. For some reason the rates are higher in the northern states, especially the northeastern states, than in the rest of the country.

For breast cancer and for most other sorts of cancer, the most important risk factor is age. Nothing else compares remotely with this in terms of predictive value. If one were to base detection efforts simply on age, one would concentrate on older women and forget the others. Looked at in terms of life expectancy and increasing life span, however, one gets a slightly different impression. Curing a woman who is 80 does not add many extra years of human life, whereas curing a woman who is 30 certainly does.

During the fall and winter of 1959, volunteer workers of the American Cancer Society persuaded over a million men and women, all over the age of 30, to answer a confidential questionnaire. Included were questions on family history, medical history, physical complaints, childbearing, and many other factors. This study was not specifically a breast cancer study. It was a general study to try to identify factors that might indicate a high or a low risk for cancer and other diseases.

The subjects were traced once a year for six years. Once every two years they were asked to answer additional question. Causes of death were ascertained from death certificates. Whenever cancer was mentioned we wrote to the doctor or to the hospital to obtain more detailed information. The data were analyzed to determine the relationship between initial factors and later occurrence of cancer.

The breast cancer death rate was more than twice as high among women whose mothers had had breast cancer as it was among those whose mothers were not recorded as having the disease. It was likewise elevated among women who reported that one or more sisters had breast cancer. Some of the subjects had a history of breast cancer before they enrolled in the study. Conceivably, female relatives had had the disease, thus leading to spurious results. Therefore, we conducted another analysis, this time excluding all subjects with a personal history of breast cancer or breast operation. The result was the same, indicating that the finding was not due to the possible bias mentioned above.

The discovery of an increased breast cancer death rate among women with family histories of the disease could indicate either of two different things. It could mean that such a family history is associated with an increased risk of developing the disease, or, alternatively, that breast cancer is more likely to be fatal among patients with such a family history. The repeat questionnaires provided a means of distinguishing between these two possibilities. The data were analyzed excluding all subjects who had a personal history of breast cancer at the time of the original questionnaire. The incidence of breast cancer, as reported on the repeat questionnaire, was about twice as high among women with a family history of the disease as among the women with a negative history. Therefore, there is an association of family history with increased incidence as distinguished from increased fatality rate.

It should be pointed out that family history data are not always reliable. This is especially so with respect to cancer which, in the not-so-distant past was an unmentionable disease. Fortunately, this attitude is changing. Because of the secrecy common in the past, many women whose mothers or sisters developed breast cancer were probably unaware of the fact. In consequence, false negative answers to questions about family history of breast cancer are probably far more common than false positive answers. Such innocent errors in reporting can result only in an underestimate in the association between family history of breast cancer and the occurrence of the disease. For this reason, I am of the opinion that family history of breast cancer is associated with the occurrence of the disease to a far greater degree than implied by the two-to-one ratio actually found. The actual relationship is probably closer to three or four to one.

The finding of familial association does not necessarily imply that the disease is inherited in the genetic sense. It might, perhaps, be inherited in a social sense of the term. Familiality is compatible with the transmittal of a virus, for example, or with environmental factors generally shared by members of a family group. The degree of association is sufficiently high to warrant investigation of these possibilities.

No matter what the explanation may be, there is a practical conclusion for the physician. If a patient has a family history of breast cancer, the physician must be doubly or quadruply alert to the possibility that she may have breast cancer herself or may develop it at some future date.

Rates of breast cancer were found to be elevated among women who had either a prior breast injury of some sort or a breast operation. This, perhaps, gives some little credence to the statement that injury may increase the rate of cancer. A different interpretation, however, seems more plausible. A relatively minor blow to the breast, which would pass unnoticed in most women, may cause pain in the cancer prone individual.

In designing the study we were hopeful that sexual history might turn out to be of some utility in detection of breast cancer or cancer of some other site. For this reason a considerable portion of the questionnaire was devoted to the subject. Breast cancer death rates were found to be approximately 40% higher in single women than in married women, but only a trifle higher in women who had not been pregnant as compared to those who had been pregnant. This is a curious combination. I am not sure what to make of it. Women whose first pregnancy occurred before the age of 25 had a lower breast cancer death rate than those whose first pregnancy occurred at an older age. The association was not great, but it was perfectly consistent. The breast cancer death rate increased slightly with advancing age at time of first pregnancy.

Age at onset of menstruation was found to be unrelated to breast cancer. Women under age 50, however, who reported irregularity in menstruation had slightly lower breast cancer death rates than other women. Late occurrence of the disease was a trifle higher among women who had had a hysterectomy than among other women. This difference was so small as to be of no significance from a practical point of view.

The taking of medicine to prevent the flow of milk showed almost no association with later occurrence of breast cancer.

I could go on at great length listing negative correlations. There are massive data on negative results. This is unfortunate but true.

The risk factors we now know are of great use to physicians in dealing with individual patients. I do not advise, however, publicizing them widely in order to bring high risk women in for detection examinations.

I was asked by a reporter a while ago, "Shouldn't we advise women with family histories of breast cancer to see their doctors?" Of course we should, but we should also advise other women to do so. The difference in risk is not great enough to warrant concentrating on a high risk group or being overly reassuring to women who have negative family histories. Telling women who have family histories of cancer to go to their doctors could be interpreted as meaning that other women do not need to go. My personal opinion is that the definition of high risk groups is useful medical information, but it should be used with caution in educational programs for the general public.

PART FOUR

MANAGEMENT OF EARLY BREAST CANCER

Breast Cancer Treatment: Change Without Improvement

WILLIAM G. HAMMOND, M.D.

Only a few years ago, there were little controlled data and less controlled research aimed at the problems of improvement in breast cancer management. Most of it was based (and still is) on the behavioral pattern typical of physicians several decades ago when presented with a woman with a mass in her breast. It was almost stereotyped behavior. "Is there really a mass in the breast? Yes, there is. I can feel it. It must be there. The patient, therefore, must come into the hospital as soon as possible, have an excisional biopsy, and, if it is positive, a radical mastectomy. If there is not really a lump there, or if I am a little different than other doctors, I may watch this for a little while, because I am not completely convinced that it has a likelihood of being cancer."

There has been a striking change since then. Now, a gynecologist, perhaps examining a woman postpartum or as part of her regular semiannual examination, may feel something in the breast and be a little unsure. He may send the patient to a general surgeon. The patient may then have mammograms. There may be a needle biopsy rather than an excisional biopsy, on the reasonably solid basis that this has not been shown to increase the hazard to the patient, that you can get a reasonably accurate diagnosis, and that it is better to have a firm tissue diagnosis before proceeding to the extensive work up that now properly precedes radical mastectomy.

Once a diagnosis of cancer is made, systemic studies must be carried out. If the patient has some skeletal pain, or if there is some radiographically suspicious area, a bone scan may be done. That may provide evidence that this patient falls within the 40% of breast cancer patients who already have systemic disease when they present themselves for treatment.

There are now a lot of things that can and often must be done. There is an abundance of research going on in many areas. There is a lot of change, but is there much improvement? I would have to say, yes, there is. The change now is at least pointing the way toward improvement. The data from the Gutmann Institute, for example, are clear. With good mammography there is earlier diagnosis, and early diagnosis should produce an increase in survival over that to which we have become accustomed. There is now a clearer understanding of the role of postoperative radiation therapy. It seems likely that it decreases local recurrence but has only a minimal impact on survival. Stjernsward, a Swedish radiotherapist, has produced some intriguing data suggesting that radiotherapy may, in fact, decrease short term survival for a select group of patients.

There is one problem that has not been settled. What is the best operation? It is suggested that so-called modified radical mastectomy may be a reasonable substitute for the classical Halsted operation, but the data that support this contention are less than solid and conflicting opinions are vocal. There is a great deal of research going on, much of it sponsored by the Breast Cancer Task Force. The definitive results, however, are not yet in. There are no hard answers regarding this most basic problem in breast cancer.

This dilemma is not unique to breast cancer. For virtually all kinds of solid tumors, the basic problem is the selection of primary management and treatment. The problem is exemplified by the facetious statement that women never die of cancer of the breast in the breast. They die of breast cancer only when it is somewhere else. Until we have reliable methods for making the diagnosis of clinically inapparent disseminated disease, there will continue to be problems with regard to treatment selection for individual patients.

The data now appearing do not show any improvement in survival with breast sparing operations. Such procedures represent improvements in the sense that the doctor can feel he is being less rough on the woman. They may represent an improvement in that the woman can feel she is more nearly normal aesthetically or physically; but none of the breast sparing operations have improved survival rates or lengthened disease free intervals when compared with radical mastectomy or its minor variants.

This can lead to an interesting speculation. How many bosoms is one woman worth? If it turns out that breast sparing operations actually decrease survivorship, the question is even more pointed. How many women is it justifiable to put at hazard of dying in the effort to spare more breasts for those who do not die?

One real improvement that might reasonably be hoped for as a result of the current atmosphere of change is a decrease in the number of polemics about equally unsatisfactory operations. Another improvement I would like very much to see is an accurate method for early diagnosis of occult metastatic spread. Still another is the development of successful therapy for occult metastasis. If enough patients were detected early with mammography and treated more promptly by surgery, this problem would decrease. It would, however, still be with us.

I would like to leave you with one interesting thought. This is the notion that there would be no urgent, compelling reason to do anything about a cancer in the breast if it were only in the breast, and if there were some reliable way to keep it from spreading while continuing evaluation. The breast mass is an indicator lesion which is more measurable and more accessible than virtually any other cancer. Since at least 40% of patients can be expected to have overt dissemination within a few years, why not see what combination chemotherapy will do to the breast lesion while it is still there, rather than remove it straightaway and lose the advantage of the indicator?

These are some of the things that I believe are worth thinking about and about which I ask you to ponder.

Surgery for Early Breast Cancer: Is There a Place for Less-Than-Radical Mastectomy? A Panel Discussion

Moderator: JEROME A. URBAN, M.D.
HENRY P. LEIS, Jr., M.D.
CONDICT MOORE, M.D.
R. WALDO POWELL, M.D.
WILLIAM W. SHINGLETON, M.D.

DR. URBAN: The detection of breast cancer when it is localized, most easily treated, and has the best prognosis is meaningless unless detection is followed by adequate treatment. During the last year there has been an aggressive publicity campaign encouraging patients with breast cancer to seek and even demand inadequate treatment for breast cancer. The rational approach to surgical treatment is being replaced by an emotional appeal to the patient. Surgery as primary treatment is being downgraded and replaced by a campaign to save the breast. This misguided wave of conservatism may well negate the tremendous potential for improved control offered by early detection, public education, and the use of more effective diagnostic aids. If we could determine the exact extent of disease reliably on initial examination, there would be no need for this panel; but we cannot. We must depend on previously developed parameters of disease behavior.

Let us begin this discussion by trying to answer some basic questions. First of all, what is the aim of surgery for primary breast cancer?

DR. POWELL: Of course, we would like to cure as many patients as possible. For practical purposes, 10 year survival with no evidence of disease is a reasonable guideline. At the same time, we would like to maintain local control, both in cured patients and in those who die of disseminated disease. Third, we would like to leave the patient cosmetically, physically, and psychologically as nearly normal as possible. Of these three aims, the first is much the most important.

DR. URBAN: We really need a definition of early breast cancer. There are a lot of different opinions about this.

DR. LEIS: The latest definition is that it is a preclinical or presymptomatic or Stage 0 breast cancer. This means a cancer that is smaller than the clinically palpable size of 1 cm, one which can only be detected by diagnostic aids. There is even a subdivision of this. Gallager has coined the phrase "minimal cancer," referring to those less than 5 mm in size. There is also early clinical cancer, Stage 1 cancer, which means a palpable lump without evidence of spread beyond the breast. Then there is the broad term "potentially curable breast cancer." This includes Stages 0, 1 and 2. Stage 2 breast cancer has involvement of the axillary nodes but no evidence of distant metastasis.

DR. URBAN: Your Stage 1 and 2 are based on clinical evaluation?

DR. LEIS: Yes.

DR. URBAN: What is the accuracy of clinical evaluation? What are its pitfalls?

DR. MOORE: Clinical evaluation is quite crude. In a number of studies comparing clinical evaluation with actual stage as determined after surgery, there is 30% error. In other words, when the axilla is clinically negative, 30% of the patients will actually have nodal involvement.

DR. URBAN: How about palpating the axilla at surgery?

DR. LEIS: This has become popular recently. Theoretically, while you are operating you can incise the pectoral fascia and palpate the axilla. This supposedly can determine whether the nodes are involved with about 70% accuracy. I must have poor fingers, because I have not been able to come even close to that accuracy. To test this, we carried out a little experiment. After finishing the dissection, we laid out the axilla, pectoral muscles, and nodes on a tray. Then the resident and I, individually, palpated and counted the number of nodes we thought we had removed and determined how many we thought were clinically involved. Our error was 23%. Even a skilled pathologist, when he sections a node and examines it grossly, cannot tell for sure whether or not it contains cancer. I am doubtful about the value of opening the axilla and palpating to determine whether metastasis is present.

DR. URBAN: A lot of the confusion in comparing statistical data is based upon clinical differences in staging. Dr. Moore, what are the factors in selecting a surgical approach? Why do we do a mastectomy? Why do we take the nodes out?

DR. MOORE: Among the factors considered when trying to tailor an operation to a particular patient, both the size of the mass and the clinical stage have influence. It is important to try to gauge the risk of a patient's having metastases in the axilla and to weigh this against the risk of removal. The relative survival is less if there are gross metastases than if there are microscopic metastases. A study done at Memorial Hospital indicated that when the nodes at the lowest level of the axilla were only microscopically involved, the eight year survival rate was 94%. When there was macroscopic involvement, that survival was cut to approximately 65%. Similarly for the mid axilla, if the nodes were only microscopically involved, the survival rate at eight years was 60%; but if they were macroscopically involved, it was about 30%.

Another important factor in picking a procedure is the possibility of multicentricity. Over half of the breasts that have cancer in them have more than one invasive site. Most importantly, if there is an insitu cancer in a breast, either lobular or ductal, 10% of those patients will have infiltrating cancer at some other focus that cannot be seen, felt, or found. This is important when considering the possibility of local excision.

DR. URBAN: Dr. Shingleton, you have gathered some rather controversial statistical material. Perhaps this is a good time to introduce it.

DR. SHINGLETON: Before that, I would like to make the basis of the controversy a little more precise. I believe that early breast cancer is not the kind of tumor that we diagnose clinically. In other malignant processes, particularly carcinoma of the cervix, it is possible to follow the cell which becomes hyperplastic and then eventually neoplastic. This may take many years. One of the striking things that has come out of epidemiologic studies that pregnancy at an early age is protective against breast cancer. Women whose first pregnancy is before age 18 have only about one-fourth the incidence of women who have their first pregnancy later. That suggests that there is something fundamental happening in the breast tissue which is related to the hormonal milieu of that patient. These facts, as well as cell kinetic studies indicate that breast cancer is a very slow growing tumor. By the time it becomes palpable, it may have existed in the breast for several years. The problem is being able to detect this breast cancer sooner so that we can treat it at some earlier stage.

So much for general thoughts. Now I will comment about some of the clinical studies related to kinds of operations. Hayward, at Guy's Hospital in London, recently published a paper surveying studies in Europe concerned with the treatment of not only early breast cancer but also of Stage 2.

McWhirter was the first maverick. Immediately after World War II, he treated a group of patients with early breast cancer by simple mastectomy and irradiation of the axilla, and compared the results with another series of patients in the same institution who had had radical mastectomy. This was not a prospective, randomized study. It is possible that the cases were selected in a different way. This is the first significant example in the modern era of a more conservative approach to treatment of early breast cancer.

A radiologist named Mustakallio in Finland used local excision of Stage 1 lesions followed by radiation of the axilla. He reported 702 patients with a 79% five year survival and a 10 year survival of 61% in 418 patients. This again was a nonrandomized study.

In this country Crile has carried out studies indicating that simple mastectomy with dissection of the axilla is as effective as radical mastectomy in Stage 1 cancer. This, too, is not a randomized study, but results were compared with those of other surgeons in the same institution who were using radical mastectomy.

Hayward has reported a survey made at the Tumor Registry of Great Britain between 1958 and 1962, comparing the results of local excision with or without irradiation, simple mastectomy, and radical mastectomy. These were all ways in which cancer of the breast was being treated in England in this four year period. There was no more than a 4% difference between one procedure and another. This, too, was not a randomized study.

Now we come to some prospective studies which have been completed. There are several still in progress. One of the first was that of Kaae and Johansen carried out in Copenhagen. They compared the McWhirter technique with extended radical mastectomy. There were 636 patients involved, and they could distinguish no difference in survival between the two groups. A study in Cambridge, England compared simple and radical mastectomy in 204 patients. Postoperative x-ray therapy was used in both groups. There was no significant difference in survival rates at five years. Hayward has now completed a prospective, randomized study at Guy's Hospital on 370 patients in both Stage 1 and Stage 2. In Stage 1 he compared "tylectomy" (excision of the local lesion) plus irradiation of the axilla with radical mastectomy. He found no significant difference in 10 year survival in patients with Stage 1 disease. In Stage 2 patients, however, there was a significant benefit in favor of radical mastectomy over local excision with irradiation of the axilla. This applied both to recurrence in the chest wall and survival.

DR. URBAN: It is important in citing these materials to realize that in a number of these studies there was a great deal of individual case selection. Five year and 10 year salvage rates are all very well, but unless you know the basis for selection of the material, you cannot understand what they mean. It is also important to know how well the patients were treated, either surgically or by radiation. There are a number of loopholes in the statistics. Dr. Leis, would you briefly enumerate the types of procedures used and briefly describe of what they consist?

DR. LEIS: Let us start with standard radical mastectomy. This includes complete removal of the breast, the pectoralis major and minor muscles, the deep pectoral fascia, the axilla, the pectoral and supramammary nodes, and the subscapular nodes. Of all the alternatives, the least extensive is simple excision, or removal of the lump. Partial mastectomy, popularized in this country by Crile is removed of 25 to 35% of the breast. It is a true partial mastectomy and leaves the patient with a smaller breast, deformed by any standard. Next in order is subcutaneous mastectomy, a shelling out of the breast. Regardless of claims to the contrary, it is not possible to remove all the breast tissue by this technique and it is not a procedure that I consider a cancer operation.

Simple mastectomy (and I hate that term) should be called total or complete mastectomy. The flaps are raised in the same way as for radical mastectomy and the dissection is carried to the same extent. It is a complete removal of the breast, and includes the axillary tail. If removal of the breast is total, an average of three to seven axillary nodes will be included. Modified radical mastectomy is a badly abused term. It may mean removal of the breast with a few axillary nodes, removal of the breast with axillary nodes or pectoral nodes, or even removal of the breast with all levels of the axillary nodes and the pectoralis minor muscle. The latter procedure is the same as the radical mastectomy except that the pectoralis major muscle is preserved. Finally, there is extended radical mastectomy, popularized by Urban.

DR. URBAN: Dr. Moore, would you talk about individualization of the approach? What factors do you consider in deciding whether to do a modified radical or some other procedure?

DR. MOORE: I consider the histology first. If the carcinoma is in situ or minimal, I use total mastectomy and remove the nodes at Level 1. If it is an invasive carcinoma, Stage 1, with no clinical suspicion of microscopic metastasis, I do a total mastectomy and an axillary dissection with or without removing the pectoralis minor but preserving the pectoralis major muscle. If the tumor is Stage 2, or if I suspect metastasis in the axilla, I do a radical mastectomy, thinking that I must rely upon surgery to remove completely any disease on the chest wall, in the breast, and in the axilla. Radiation therapy can be added to deal with the supraclavicular and the internal mammary nodes.

I have not mentioned the risk of internal mammary node metastasis. That risk is high in lesions in the inner half of the breast. Both Urban and Handley have shown by biopsies that there are metastases in the internal mammary nodes in about half of the patients with medial lesions and that the metastases are often microscopic. One has to take this into account and treat these nodes in one way or another. I have chosen, in recent years, to use post-operative radiotherapy, and I think that it has produced fair rate of control, although perhaps not as great as that Urban has obtained with extended radical mastectomy.

DR. URBAN: Dr. Leis, will you bring us up to date on current survival statistics? Then we will discuss a few patients.

DR. LEIS: I am fascinated by the figures that are being thrown around. Obviously, only 10 year survival rates should be used as a basis for comparisons. For lumpectomy, Crile's figures show a 10 year survival of 34.4%. While this rate is said to apply to Stage 1 and Stage 2 cancers, the series must have been heavily weighted with Stage 1. In Miller's report of a group treated by simple mastectomy, Stage 1 and Stage 2 cases, the 10 year survival rate is 36%. In Handley's report of a modified radical mastectomy series, the rate is 50%. At the Cleveland Clinic, when they combined simple and modified radicals, a 10 year survival rate of 41% was achieved. The lowest rate reported with radical mastectomy, that of the National Breast Cancer Group, is 42.8%. The highest, reported from Memorial Hospital, actually a combined radical and extended radical mastectomy series, is 61%. The average, from many different published series, for radical mastectomy is between 53 and 56%. There is clearly a big difference between lesser procedures and more extensive procedures.

I do not want to give the impression that I favor doing the same procedure for everybody. A procedure should be selected to fit the patient. For noninvasive cancers, I do simple mastectomy. For Stage 0 presymptomatic cancers found by mammography, I do a simple mastectomy with low axillary dissection. For adenoid cystic carcinoma, medullary carcinoma with lymphoid stroma, tubular carcinoma, mucinous carcinoma, and papillary carcinoma, I prefer the true modified radical mastectomy, as Handley has popularized it. For the common infiltrating, scirrhous carcinoma, the most common cancer we have, one must make a choice between modified radical and radical mastectomy. Extended radical mastectomy is appropriate for medial or central lesions. A modified radical or radical mastectomy in this situation requires postoperative radiation. This is the only area in which there is much controversy.

DR. URBAN: I would like to ask the panel how they would treat this patient. She is 45 years of age and has superficial Paget's disease in the right breast. There is no palpable mass beneath the nipple. Deep wedge biopsy showed Paget's disease and noninfiltrating cancer in the underlying ducts.

DR. MOORE: Studies have shown that when there is no mass to be felt in Paget's disease, there is hardly ever a metastasis in the axilla. I think total mastectomy would be adequate treatment for this.

DR. LEIS: We have been caught short a few times with Paget's disease that did not seem to have any palpable mass. In these cases, we do total mastectomy with axillary gland dissection, and we have occasionally been surprised to find in some other segment of the breast a small infiltrating cancer. I agree, however, that this is rare.

DR. URBAN: Probably a nice approach would be to do a modified radical mastectomy and have the nodes checked. If they are negative that would be fine. If there were extensive nodal disease in the axilla and a central infiltrating cancer, there would be a strong probability of internal mammary node metastasis. I think, however, that we can agree that this is a favorable patient who could be treated adequately by modified radical mastectomy. The second patient is in her early forties. The tumor was evident by x-ray and physical examination, and biopsy showed a low grade malignant cystosarcoma.

DR. SHINGLETON: I believe that this is a fairly favorable lesion. I would do a total mastectomy, but I would do a lymph node dissection along with it.

DR. URBAN: What would you expect to find in the axilla? What is the risk of finding nodal disease?

DR. SHINGLETON: In my experience, it has been quite low.

DR. URBAN: Theoretically, you might interfere with the protective mechanism by removing lymph nodes. This might be far more dangerous than leaving disease there.

DR. SHINGLETON: I agree that the nodes may be signals. The lesion, however, has been present for years and if there are no signals present at the time of operation, it's not likely that they will appear postoperatively.

DR. LEIS: These cystosarcomas are not necessarily true sarcomas. They can have a carcinomatous component, and by leaving nodes behind, you can miss this.

DR. URBAN: Right! In our experience 3% of these patients have nodes in the axilla. The opposite breast of the patient looked and felt completely normal.

DR. SHINGLETON: Did you have a mammogram taken of it?

DR. URBAN: Yes, we did. This is the whole point. When there is a malignant neoplasm in one breast, it is a good idea to have a mammogram to evaluate the opposite side. This patient happened to have an 8 mm infiltrating carcinoma at twelve o'clock.

DR. SHINGLETON: This was visible by mammogram?

DR. URBAN: Yes, but not palpable. How would you handle this?

DR. SHINGLETON: I would use the same procedure as on the opposite breast, total mastectomy for an early invasive tumor.

DR. URBAN: She had a bilateral modified radical mastectomy and is free of disease. The third patient has a mass 2.5 cm in diameter in the upper inner quadrant, and biopsy shows infiltrating duct cancer. The axilla is equivocal.

DR. LEIS: With centrally or medially located lesions, the incidence of internal mammary lymph node involvement is high. To achieve local control, you must either do an extended radical mastectomy or use the standard radical mastectomy and give radiation to both the internal mammary chains. The latter would be my preference, although the extended radical would also be an excellent approach.

DR. URBAN: Thank you. To sum up, we believe it is best to attempt to remove all disease present in the breast and the regional nodes. This should always be tempered by the extent of disease present in the patient.

What the Plastic Surgeon Has to Offer in the Management of Breast Tumors

REUVEN K. SNYDERMAN, M.D.

What the plastic surgeon has to offer in the management of breast tumors is simple: it is hope. It is hope for the patient that, after having had her tumor removed, she can be restored not as she was, but at least to something she can accept. The female breast means many things to many people, but in American society today it is, of course, a sex symbol. By modern methods, satisfactory reconstruction can be achieved. We cannot make every patient look perfect, but as plastic surgeons we do have something to offer.

Breast reconstruction is not new. The older method was basically that of migrating massive amounts of tissue from somewhere else on the body. Many stages were necessary. The time required frequently ran from a year to a year and one-half. By the time the procedure was finished, the patient usually was fed up both with the process and with the doctor.

In recent years, the use of implantable material for augmentation of the human breast has made possible a new method of reconstruction. This procedure is also used for the woman with asymmetrical breasts who is unhappy and unable to wear proper clothes. By the use of a silicone implant placed behind the breast, we can in this situation produce a near normal appearance.

From this we have learned how to make use of the silicones. The improvement in implants that has taken place over the last 20 years has made it possible for us not only to offer this group of women some improvement, but also to restore contour for those who have undergone mastectomies, even with the loss of pectoral muscles. The companies are working with us. They will make prostheses to practically any design we desire. Remember that what we are doing in the reconstruction of the female breast is by no means a cosmetic triumph. What we are aiming for is to allow women to look decent in clothes. This seems to be especially important to young women, who often feel that the wearing of an external prosthesis is difficult and that they will be exposed by wearing a bathing suit or tennis dress.

Another breast problem in which we plastic surgeons are interested is that of the woman who has had multiple breast masses, who has had multiple biopsies, and who is living with the constant fear that the next one is going to prove to be malignant. In this situation, we carry out subcutaneous mastectomy, which is an attempt to remove most of the breast tissue. After approximately six months, the skin has softened and then an implant can be put in. The same procedure can be applied to lesions such as in situ lobular carcinoma. I am not saying this is a cancer operation. It definitely is not. But in the situation where the woman refuses mastectomy, it is one way of gaining some measure of patient cooperation. Both breasts should be done at the same time.

In doing subcutaneous mastectomy, we start with an inframammary incision and work up to the fascia behind the pectoralis muscles. Then we start the dissection up under the skin. There may be difficult spots at the sites of old biopsies and behind the nipple. Here the dissection must be carried extremely close to the skin. Once the entire mass of the breast is freed and the dissection has been continued into the axillary area as far as possible, the entire breast tissue is removed.

In the early days, we inserted the prosthesis immediately. This is a silicone bag filled with liquid silicon. The shape and contour as well as the texture have been improved over the years. More recently, however, because of an occasional slough of tissue, we have elected first to do the subcutaneous mastectomy, as carefully as possible, then to wait for approximately six months until the skin softens, and then to insert the implant.

It is important when considering subcutaneous mastectomy to plan to do both breasts at the same time. There are two reasons for this. First, the lesions for which this operation is appropriate have a high probability of being bilateral, even if the bilaterality is not clinically apparent. Second, it is extremely difficult to attain the desired degree of symmetry under these circumstances with a unilateral prosthesis.

One other point to be emphasized is that the subcutaneous mastectomy specimen must be sent to the laboratory and meticulously examined by the pathologist, with x-ray control, to look for any suspicious areas.

Reconstruction after mastectomy is based on similar principles, but presents some added problems. Those ugly mastectomy scars once so common are fast disappearing. My general surgical colleagues assure me that this type of wound and incision is no longer necessary. Any type of scar, however, introduces additional difficulties.

Most women who have had mastectomies adjust by the end of six months. If they fail to do so, they should be given the opportunity of at least discussing with a plastic surgeon what can be done. Out of every 100 women with whom I go through this sort of discussion, only about 5% ultimately decide to undergo the surgery once they have found out what is available and what it will require. Some are satisfied with less than complete procedures, such as the simple formation of a mound. They no longer have to wear an external prosthesis.

Complete reconstruction, if it is to be carried out, can begin about six months after mastectomy. Because the skin is only slightly movable over the chest wall, a small prosthesis is first inserted. After a period of time, enough stretching of the skin occurs that a larger prosthesis can be substiuted. Of course, the scar may need to be improved. Some can be and some cannot. We can also produce an areola and nipple, but this may be more than the patient desires. Once the implant is inserted, she may be satisfied with the fact that she can buy a normal bra and wear normal clothes. The aim is for the patient to look normal and natural when she has clothes on her body. It may be necessary to reduce the other breast to bring it into better alignment with the reconstructed breast. In fact, many women with large breasts may be benefited by this procedure alone.

There are many other things we can do for these patients. We can revise the scar, take out a dog ear, or even, if it is desired, by a minor procedure create something that resembles a nipple.

There has been some discussion about saving the nipple when a mastectomy is done. This can be accomplished by transplanting it to an adjacent region, provided very careful dissection is made beneath it and the tissue is sent to the pathologist. If the subareolar tissue is reported to be invaded, the transplanted nipple is immediately removed. I see no real reason for having the backup nipple when a satisfactory substitute can be constructed by less risky means.

Let us briefly go over again the uses of the subcutaneous mastectomy. I think this procedure is indicated (a) when three or more previous biopsies have been carried out, (b) when there is a family hisory of breast cancer, (c) in a woman who is psychologically obsessed to the point of being unable to function each time she finds a new mass, (d) following mastectomy for removal of the other breast, and (e) for carcinoma, when other types of treatment have been refused. Subcutaneous mastectomy is not to be used for carcinoma when other methods of treatment are available.

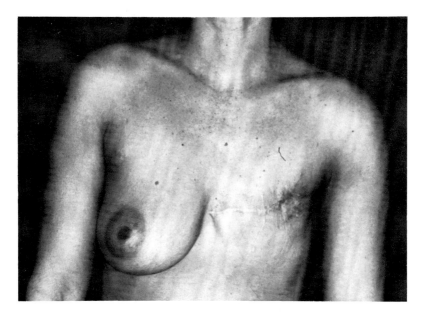

Figure 1. Case 1. Preoperative appearance.

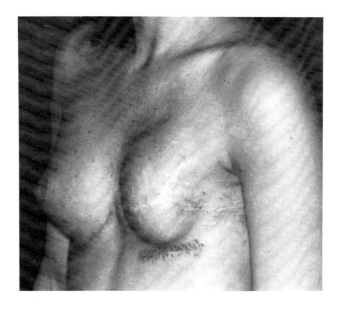

Figure 2. Case 1. Appearance after creation of a left breast by silicone implant and reduction mammoplasty on the right for equalization.

From the standpoint of the plastic surgeon, the steps to follow after mastectomy are (a) conduct a full and frank discussion with the patient, (b) provide help in rehabilitation, either directly in some circumstances, or through the Reach for Recovery program, (c) make sure the patient has a properly fitting prosthesis, and (d) if she is still unhappy, send her to discuss the matter with a plastic surgeon.

What does the plastic surgeon have to offer to the patient who has had a mastectomy? We can reduce a large breast, we can create a mound on the mastectomy side by inserting a prosthesis, we can create an areola and a nipple, and we can revise scars. Most important, we can offer hope to the woman who finds mastectomy impossible to bear.

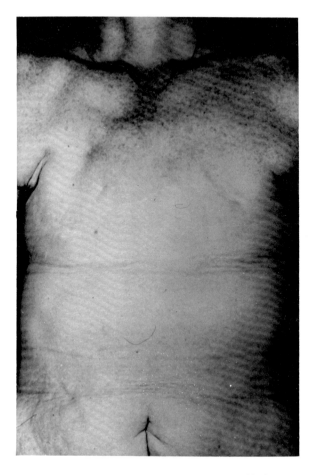

Figure 3.   Case 2. Appearance after bilateral mastectomy and before reconstruction.

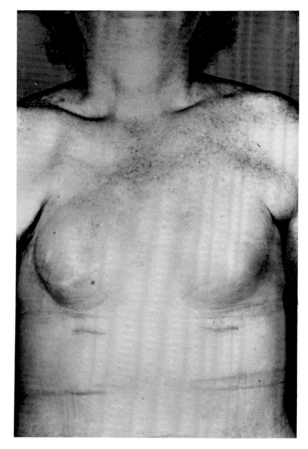

Figure 4. Case 2. Silicone implants have been placed bilaterally.

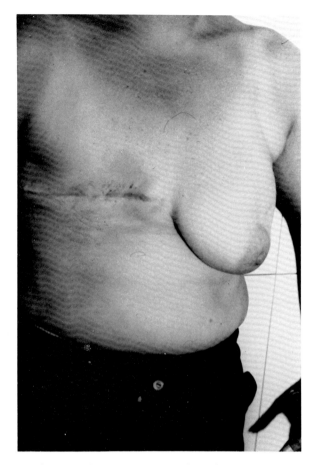

Figure 5. Case 3. Appearance after right mastectomy.

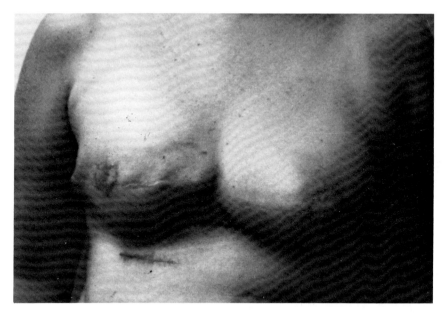

Figure 6. Case 3. A right breast has been formed by a silicone implant. The left breast has been reduced in size and excess areola from the left has been used to create a new areola on the right.

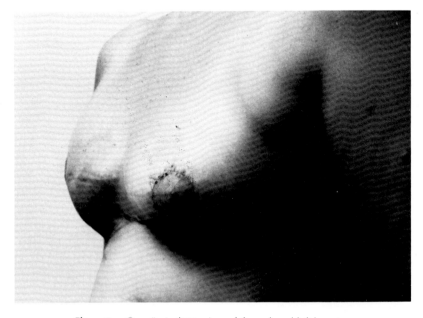

Figure 7. Case 3. A closer view of the reduced left breast.

138

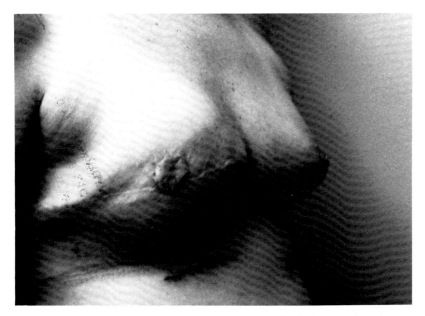

Figure 8.   Case 3. Detailed view of the reconstructed right breast and areola.

What We Have Learned and Are Learning from Cooperative Clinical Trials

BERNARD FISHER, M.D.

F requently, I am asked why we need randomized, prospective clinical trials? What is the matter with retrospective information? This is an important question. Retrospective data have given us much. More and more, however, clinicians are becoming aware that conclusions reached in a retrospective fashion are based on data that were not originally gathered to answer the questions asked of it. More than that, it is frequently difficult to be sure of the equality of the groups compared using retrospective data. There are nothing wrong with retrospective data, but it is wrong to ascribe more credibility to retrospective data than they deserve.

Retrospective data give suggestive evidence. They are like laboratory experimentation in which one laboratory does an experiment on one animal model system and another laboratory uses another. If enough animal model systems demonstrate a certain phenomenon, we then must say to ourselves, "Well, this looks promising. We will have to find out what happens in man." It is similar with retrospective data. Retrospective data give us suggestive information, but it is only through the clinical trial mechanism that one can obtain definitive answers.

Beginning in 1958, there was established what has now become known as the National Surgical Adjuvant Breast Project. The purpose was to evaluate, through a prospective randomized approach, certain modalities in the treatment of primary breast cancer. I would like to describe briefly some of the things the NSABP has accomplished and also some of the problems encountered with these clinical trials.

First, we have gotten people to begin to realize that breast cancer is not purely a surgical problem. By the clinical trial mechanism, radiation therapists, surgeons, and medical oncologists have begun to talk to each other.

One of the interesting things that has come from these studies over the last 10 years is valid information about the results of radical mastectomy in this country. It is all very well for one individual or one group to report results. It is equally important, however, that we know as closely as we can, what the results are for this operation in the country as a whole. The NSABP results indicate that the overall treatment failure rate is 49.5% within 10 years. For all patients with positive nodes it is 76%. In negative node patients there is a 24% treatment failure rate. Patients with one to three positive nodes have a 65% treatment failure rate and in those with four or more positive nodes it is 86%.

This demonstrates several things. First, it indicates that what happens by 5 years is a good indication of what is going to happen in 10 years. There is gradual regression of the survival curve, but the bulk of the failures occur within the first 5 years following mastectomy.

The overall survival rate at 10 years in this group of patients is 45.9%. For all positive node patients it is 24.9%. For patients with four or more positive nodes, it is 13.4%. For those with one to three positive nodes it is 37%.

The variation in the number of nodes removed at radical mastectomy is tremendous, as one might expect. This may be due to surgical variation, pathologist variation, or perhaps to anatomical variation in women. The number of nodes removed, however, has no influence on the treatment failure rate. This is true for both negative and positive node patients.

In these prospective studies, it has been demonstrated that less than 2% of patients developed a secondary primary carcinoma within six years.

We have concluded that it is categorically possible to make the statement that results are related to tumor size, but this alone is not the answer. Patients with extremely small tumors and positive axillary nodes do less well than patients with large tumors and no involvement of axillary nodes.

We have also published information relative to the effect of location of the tumor. The results of these studies demonstrated no difference ascribable to the location of tumor, whether inner or outer quadrant. The results were the same when the treatment was radical mastectomy.

The original purpose of this clinical trial was to determine whether adjunct chemotherapy given at the time of surgery and postoperatively would have any beneficial effect. We did not find any effect in general. In one subgroup, premenopausal patients with four or more positive nodes, there was a delay of 16 months in treatment failure time. The important thing is that we were able to answer this question in a relatively short period of time. Without the trial, we still would have no answer.

On postoperative radiation therapy following radical mastectomy, I can only quote the results. I do not intend to editorialize. There was no increase in survival of patients receiving postoperative radiation therapy over the control group. This was true in all the patient groups. There was some effect upon local recurrence. In the placebo group, 15% had local recurrence. This was reduced to 8% with radiation therapy. The incidence of internal mammary and supraclavicular node recurrence was 3% in the placebo group; following radiation therapy, it was less than 1%. It is important to put the magnitude of these reductions in proper prospective. It may very well be that radiation administered in this trial was inadequate or inappropriate. But, this was the kind of radiation therapy that was being given to patients all over this country at that particular time.

We did a prospective, randomized clinical trial to determine whether surgical castration would have any effect if done after mastectomy, and it did not. There was no evidence that prophylactic castration had any advantage.

There is now in progress a large prospective, randomized clinical study to accumulate firm data to determine whether total mastectomy with radiation is equivalent to radical mastectomy. Here we randomize the patients according to whether they have clinically positive or negative axillary nodes. We have enrolled 1450 patients in this study in two and one-half years. Over 200 surgeons from more than 30 institutions are participating. When total mastectomy is done and positive axillary nodes develop subsequently, we want to find out whether delayed axillary dissection is equivalent to immediate axillary dissection. We want to know if radiation following total mastectomy is as good as radical mastectomy and whether one can sterilize the axillary nodes in positive axillary node patients.

The most remarkable thing about this is that this is not a surgical trial only. There is pathologist and radiotherapist involvement. People are getting together to try to get an answer in as short a time as possible, and not 100 years from now.

What we find in this trial will indicate whether a trial of segmental mastectomy should be done. There is today no evidence to support the contention that segmental mastectomy is as good as or better than radical mastectomy. If we find that total mastectomy with radiation produces results better than or equivalent to radical mastectomy, then, logically, the next step would be to do a trial of total mastectomy with radiation versus segmental mastectomy with radiation. On the other hand, if our present trial shows that radical mastectomy is, indeed, better than total mastectomy with radiation, there is no justification for considering a clinical trial of segmental mastectomy. Similarly, if total mastectomy alone is better than or equivalent to radical mastectomy, then we should proceed to a trial of total mastectomy alone versus the segmental mastectomy alone. If we show that total mastectomy is not as good as radical mastectomy, then there is no reason to do this kind of trial.

There are other trials now being contemplated, using combination chemotherapy, immunotherapy, and other modalities. Only if these trials can be made can answers be obtained quickly. Valid answers can only be obtained if one can really assure oneself that he is comparing, as nearly as is humanly possible, two equivalent groups of patients. That is what the clinical trial mechanism is all about.

One of the major problems in carrying out clinical trials is the difficulty of enlisting physician participation. Clinical trials are a science, and to many clinicians they are incomprehensible. This includes internists, radiation therapists, medical oncologists, and surgeons. It includes young men and old, and those from prestigious institutions as well as those in private practice.

For several generations, the trend in medical education has been to stress individualism, particularly as it relates to therapeutic decision making. Now we are asking the clinician to condition himself in the opposite direction. Decisions are made for him by clinical trials. He feels that this infringes on his right to determine "proper" therapy or to individualize therapy, and for such reasons he cannot participate.

Another reason for nonparticipation is related to the referring physician. By the very nature of our system of health care delivery in this country, referring physicians are frequently in the position of influencing medical practice. The surgeon fears that if he randomizes, the selection will not coincide with the expectations of the referring physician.

Another significant problem is the trauma of communication with the patient to obtain informed consent, which is mandatory. This necessitates more dialogue between the patient and surgeon than ordinarily may occur. Many surgeons would just as soon avoid the resultant tension and anxiety and sidestep participation. It has been our overwhelming experience that when the evaluation is properly explained to a patient, she is anxious to become involved and is more cooperative in follow-up. When patients have refused to cooperate, it can usually be traced to the way in which the program was presented to them.

There are other problems. There are surgical residents who feel that their best interests are not met by clinical trials. All sorts of problems are encountered in doing clinical trials. But the ready acceptance of the prospective, randomized clinical trial is one of the major medical advances of our time.

Response to Demands for Patient Participation in Treatment Selection: A Panel Discussion

Moderator: ARTHUR I. HOLLEB, M.D.
LAMAN A. GRAY, M.D.
CHARLES W. HAYDEN, M.D.
ELEANOR D. MONTAGUE, M.D.
REUVEN K. SNYDERMAN, M.D.

DR. HOLLEB: Now more than ever before, patients have become health oriented consumers. They read newspapers and magazines, hear radio programs, and see television shows about breast cancer. Some of the reporting is excellent and some, unfortunately, emphasizes controversy. The Gallup poll has shown us how poorly educated, if not abysmally ignorant, American people are about breast cancer. Women are marching on clinics and private offices waving copies of *McCall's, Good Housekeeping, Ms., Playgirl,* or the supplement of their local newspaper, advising doctors about quotations from Crile, Cope, Nolan, Urban, Anglem, Robbins, Leis, and others. They are quoting statistics. They are asking questions using technical terms such as tylectomy, lumpectomy, standard radical, extended radical, and so on.

Occasionally one hears statements such as "Surgeons are male chauvinists determined to deprive women of their femininity." Or, "Physicians are inflexible in their approach to breast cancer. They have not changed in 40 years." Or, "I have the right to decide whether I keep my breast or lose it."

Let me ask the panel this: What are your thoughts about the way the media have handled information about breast cancer?

DR. MONTAGUE: The consternation reflected in the media has been brought about by the actions of physicians themselves. In the last 25 years or so, there has been a lack of conversation with and sympathy for patients. Too many patients get too little information from their doctors, and if they do not get information from their doctors they are going to get it somewhere. The media have stepped into that void.

DR. HAYDEN: We have gone from a comfortable, static position to one of uncomfortable changeability, and the media have been responsible for this. I personally have welcomed the furor because it has made me more aware of my inadequacy to answer the logical questions that patients bring up.

DR. SNYDERMAN: The main problem over the years has been that doctors would not talk to reporters, so newsmen have gone elsewhere to get what they desired. As qualified people become more willing to talk, better articles will be written.

DR. GRAY: The sensationalism of some of the articles has raised hackles among my colleagues. On the other hand, some of the coverage has been pretty well done by the press. An article that appeared in the *Memphis Commercial Appeal* a week ago is really very good. It tells a great deal that people need to know, and includes a great deal to stir the medical profession.

DR. HOLLEB: Obviously no surgical or radiotherapeutic procedure can be performed without the patient having signed a consent form. How meaningful is this document? What is the relevance of informed consent?

DR. MONTAGUE: The majority of consent forms I have seen do not provide much information to the patient. A signature on a piece of paper is relatively easy to obtain, especially from patients of low educational level. With the advent of the clinical trials, though, this is changing, and consent is more generally truly informed consent. The patient gets the full description of the study from a physician. We spend more time talking about the informed consent than we do about any other aspect of the treatment. This change has taken place largely though the efforts of Dr. Fisher and the NSABP and it is nationwide.

DR. SNYDERMAN: The consent form can never portray what you really mean. What is important is that the patient understand, within her ability to understand, exactly what you have in mind. You have to give her a chance to talk back to you. You may be worrying about some protocol, and she may be interested in some simple, little thing like "When can I go home?" or "Do I have to come back to your office to have the sutures removed?" If she is not given a chance to verbalize this, she feels she has not been given a chance to express her fears and doubts. If this communication gap can be bridged, much of the distrust caused by articles in the press can be negated.

DR. HAYDEN: I explain definitely to every woman with a breast tumor what I plan to do. Previously it was no problem. Now you have to be more specific about how much of that breast you are going to remove.

DR. GRAY: Our hospital is one of the few in the country that does not have a signed permission for operation. Every surgeon, however, must explain the procedure carefully to his patient and make a note in the chart that he has explained to her what he intends to do and what the various options are.

DR. HOLLEB: Dr. Hayden, your time is pretty well occupied. How much time do you actually spend with a patient in discussing what is going to be done?

DR. HAYDEN: Not a great deal until I have something definitive to talk about. That is why it's important to get something in the way of a biopsy report promptly. Then we can explain what we plan to do and why.

DR. HOLLEB: Dr. Montague, at the M. D. Anderson Hospital you have a surgeon, a radiotherapist, and an internist all dealing with the patient almost simultaneously. How does this work in terms of discussing with the individual what may be done?

DR. MONTAGUE: This is the only practical method of supplying to the patient the multidisciplinary environment necessary for breast cancer treatment. We have passed beyond the period when a patient belonged to one clinician. Regardless of the environment, nowadays a physician is never really by himself. Breast cancer is one of the most complicated of cancers to treat, and good management requires more than one opinion. In our institution, the patient is examined prior to biopsy or definitive treatment by a surgeon, a radiotherapist, and an internist, because all of these people are going to participate in her care at some point. It is distinctly advantageous for the medical oncologist to see the patient when she is well.

At M. D. Anderson Hospital, the physician who does the explaining to the patient is the one whom the group decides will have the main control of her treatment. If the decision of the group is for a radical mastectomy, then the explanation will come from the surgeon. If, on the other hand, the patient has had her surgery and is coming in for postoperative radiation therapy, the surgeon sees her and so does the medical oncologist. The discussion, however, will come from the radiation therapist.

DR. HOLLEB: Dr. Snyderman, as a plastic surgeon do you see patients preoperatively and postoperatively?

DR. SNYDERMAN: Unfortunately, I do not see enough of them before their mastectomies. Particularly for patients who are extremely fearful, it is reassuring to have a preoperative conversation with a plastic surgeon. The most frequent complaint of women who come to me after mastectomy is that their surgeons have not talked to them. The patient finds a lump. She goes to a surgeon's office. He finds a lump. He calls the secretary and says, "Book her tomorrow." The next thing she knows she is in the hospital, has had a biopsy, and has had her breast off. And this is all the communication that went on. Now, maybe this is not altogether true. Maybe the woman was so frightened at that original visit that she did not listen. But it is from the physician that help must come, and if it takes time, you just have to find it.

DR. MONTAGUE: Most of the patients I see come because their surgeons have refused to discuss with them alternative treatments or even the possibility of having a biopsy done prior to making a treatment decision. Many patients do not mind the prospect of radical mastectomy. They do not mind having any procedure that is recommended. But they do mind going into the hospital and having both procedures done under the same anesthesia. A little bit of talking often eliminates the problem. There are, however, many patients, and they are increasing in number, who want to wake up after the biopsy and find out what the treatment is going to be, rather than wake up in the recovery room and feel around to see what the treatment has been. This is going to be a real problem in the future, and I think it is about time that the problem is recognized.

DR. HAYDEN: I agree. In fact, I have changed my procedures to fit in with what Dr. Montague is saying. I try to shorten the interval between the detection of the lump and definitive diagnosis. Needle aspiration solves approximately 80% of my problems, because about 80% are simple benign cysts. In the case of a small lump in a small breast I do a local excision in the office. This takes care of another 10%. The remainder must go to the hospital, but we are finding that the in-out patient concept can shorten the time considerably.

DR. HOLLEB: Has there been any change that you have noticed in patient participation, or in acceptance or rejection of this approach?

DR. HAYDEN: Patients are happier with it. These women want to participate and want to know what can be done.

DR. HOLLEB: Dr. Hayden, how often do you see women who do not want to know anything about what you are going to do; who do not want to be bothered with facts, details, or descriptions?

DR. HAYDEN: The majority of them are like that. A few women are obsessed with the idea that you have to treat them with absolute openness and explain everything, but at present they constitute only a trickle. I am anticipating that there are going to be more, and I am trying to prepare myself for that onslaught.

DR. HOLLEB: Does anybody have an instruction sheet or booklet to be given to patients before they enter the hospital? Should there be one? Is it better not to have one because of variations in circumstances?

DR. HAYDEN: I use a booklet prepared by Dr. Leis and it is very helpful. I think that Memorial Hospital has one also. This is where you begin to lay the

groundwork for the phase of rehabilitation, the problems of possible reconstruction, the remaining breast, and recurrence. These are problems in
which patient participation is really necessary.

DR. HOLLEB: Let us get down to specific situations. Dr. Synderman, suppose a 40 year old woman came to you with a diagnosis of lobular carcinoma
in situ. She has been advised by a general surgeon to have a mastectomy, but
she has refused. In your relationship with her what would you tell her? What
would you do surgically, if anything?

DR. SNYDERMAN: I would discuss once again with her what had been advised, and I would agree that she should have a mastectomy. I would also try
to find out if there had been a personality clash between this patient and the
surgeon she saw originally. If the patient continued to be adamant, I would
ask her to consult one other breast surgeon. Then, if the circumstances did
not change, I would do a subcutaneous mastectomy. Doing something for
her is better than having her wander off and receive inadequate treatment
or none at all.

DR. HOLLEB: Suppose she had had an invasive carcinoma?

DR. SNYDERMAN: The same thing. If the woman refuses everything else,
subcutaneous mastectomy is better than nothing.

DR. MONTAGUE: If the patient refuses definitive surgical treatment, I believe it is important for her physician to realize that there are other methods
of treatment. We radiotherapists get patients who have had all kinds of
procedures, all kinds of biopsies, all kinds of surgery. We treat the patient no
matter what. All we want is a positive tissue diagnosis. If the tumor is small
and the patient refuses even to have an excision (and that is very rare), we
can treat it with radiation therapy, and we can tell her that her chances are
quite good.

DR. HOLLEB: Suppose a personal friend of yours were discovered to have a
1 cm carcinoma and had been advised to have a radical mastectomy by a
general surgeon. Would you try to dissuade her from having it done?

DR. MONTAGUE: No. Never.

DR. HOLLEB: Does anybody on the panel feel that need for the help of a
psychiatrist in dealing with the patients who have had mastectomies recommended?

DR. HAYDEN: I do not.

DR. SNYDERMAN: A psychiatrist should examine some of the patients, but
when you suggest it, the first comment is "What do you think I am, crazy?"
There are not enough psychiatrists who are willing to undertake this sort of
problem on the basis of one or two visits.

DR. HOLLEB: How about other members of the family? Should they be
involved preoperatively and postoperatively in discussions?

DR. HAYDEN: The husband is the one we find it necessary to include most often. The others are involved more from the standpoint of family history and risk.

DR. HOLLEB: Many of us have a tendency to talk about individualizing patients. What exactly does this mean? How do you go about indiviudalizing patients?

DR. MONTAGUE: The term "individualize" is not a good one for the kind of patient selection of which I am in favor. I think that there is little logical patient selection throughout the country. The majority of patients have their surgery with only meager preoperative examinations and rarely any diagrams or descriptions of grave signs. You might say that the M. D. Anderson plan is individualization, but it is not. Rather, there is a framework of treatment into which patients can fit.

DR. HAYDEN: The essence of my approach has been careful selectivity. This is especially important in deciding what to do about the remaining breast.

QUESTION: Don't you think you get better results if you discuss all the alternatives and try to make the patient understand the treatment selected, even if the patient says, "Doctor, do anything you want. I just want to get well"?

DR. MONTAGUE: The question of how much to tell the patient is bounded by the limits of practicality. It would take two hours to talk about all of the various possibilities related to the simplest procedure. Rather than going into tremendous detail, if the physician can approach the patient with kindness and sympathy and with an attentive ear, if he will listen to what the patient is trying to tell him, he can do a great deal. The principal thing is sympathy and empathy with the patient.

DR. HOLLEB: Our time is up. I should like to express my appreciation to the members of the panel for being so patient with me and also to the audience for its close attention.

Preoperative Radiographic Localization of Nonpalpable Lesions

GERALD D. DODD, M.D.

Everyone agrees that the ultimate aim and the greatest benefit of mammography is the detection of clinically occult lesions. This places on the radiologist not only the responsibility of making the diagnosis but also that of making certain that the surgeon is directed to the proper region of the breast from which to obtain representative tissue. Furthermore, once the biopsy has been done, the radiologist must make sure that, indeed, the tissue in question has been removed, and that the pathologist is directed to the part of the specimen that requires histologic examination. Most frequently this problem arises when there are small calcific deposits in the breast, but it can also occur with small nonpalpable soft tissue densities.

I would like to describe a case that sums up the difficulties that can result from failure to pay close attention to every detail in this process. A 62 year old woman came for mammography at her own request. She was referred by her doctor with some reluctance. She had no clinical findings. The mammograms showed a large calcium deposit, almost certainly a calcified fibroadenoma. A little distance away, however, was a cluster of tiny flecks of calcium. We reported a possible carcinoma in the upper medial quadrant. The surgeon felt nothing and at first was unwilling to operate. After considerable persuasion, however, he acquiesced. He wisely took the mammograms to the operating room, but unwisely did not take the radiologist. The result was that the histologic examination was negative. When I asked the surgeon if he had encountered any calcium, he replied, "There was a lot. I got the area. It was not a cancer. And the whole thing was a farce."

It took approximately six weeks after the patient was discharged from the hospital for me to talk the surgeon into sending her back for another mammogram. Sure enough, the large calcium deposit was gone, but the tiny flecks in the upper medial quadrant remained, 2 or 3 cm from the biopsy site. The surgeon was upset when we told him that he had missed the cancer. He then provided us with a biopsy that was almost a subcutaneous mastectomy. A specimen radiograph found the calcium we were looking for, and histologically it proved to be due to a small intraductal carcinoma.

I am as critical of myself in this case as I am of the surgeon; in fact more so. I did not localize the important lesion for him. I did not go over the films during our discussions and I did not send adequate information to the operating room. As a result, the patient had to have two surgical procedures, and finally a third, since radical mastectomy was subsequently done.

If one approaches this kind of situation with forethought, errors can be avoided. Berger, Gershon-Cohen, and Isard in 1966 described one effective method for localization of nonpalpable lesions. What they did was place the cephalocaudad and lateral x-ray views adjacent to a piece of paper on which were diagrammed views of the breast as seen from above, laterally and frontally. Lines were drawn through the nipple, dividing the breast into quadrants. The area in question was projected onto the diagram. This diagram can be sent to the operating room to provide clearly stated information as to the quadrant in which the tumor lies, the diameter of the suspect area, and the depth of the deposit below the skin. The authors emphasize that it is absolutely necessary that the patient be positioned on the operating table in such a way that the projected lines through the nipple are approximately the same as those in the diagram. Under these circumstances, this is a highly accurate way of localizing the suspect tissue. Needless to say, specimen radiography must be done.

Recently, in some unpublished work, Dr. Gloria Frankel of Los Angeles described a modification of this. The lesion is first located as to quadrant. Dr. Frankel then places a strip of plastic numbers along each boundary of the quadrant in question and reradiographs the breast. She locates the suspicious area with respect to the numbers in both views and marks the sites of the closest numbers with silver nitrate. The surgeon can use these two points to triangulate the location of the tissue in question.

Both of these techniques are reasonably accurate, but they require the excision of at least one quadrant of the breast to make sure that all of the area of the lesion is included in the specimen. Since most of these small lesions turn out to be benign, we would prefer to disfigure the breast as little as possible. There is a way to accomplish this, even though it is a little more time consuming.

We start with a diagram of the breast which is a modification of that of Berger, Gershon-Cohen, and Isard. The suspect area is merely projected roughly into a quadrant of the breast. We do not send the diagram to the operating room, however, but bring the patient to the radiology department an hour or so prior to the surgical procedure. She is positioned just as she was for the original mammograms. Then, using the diagram, we insert one or more needles into the lesion. A radiograph is taken to determine if we have approximated the area in question. Any needle not properly positioned is removed. The patient is then sent to the operating room with the needle or needles in place. All the surgeon has to do is to remove a core of tissue around the needle and send it to the laboratory for the usual specimen radiograph and frozen section.

This has proved to be highly accurate. It is not really necessary to transfix the mass or the deposit as long as the relationship between the position of the needle and that of the lesion can be relayed to the surgeon. As a matter of fact, in patients with large breasts, we do not attempt to go into the middle at all, but simply place the needle point at the periphery of the calcium deposit. It is then only necessary to indicate to the surgeon that if the material within 2 to 3 cm of the point is taken, he should encompass the lesion.

By this method we avoid the deformity resulting from removal of a large amount of tissue yet still secure an accurate histologic diagnosis. This procedure is more precise than attempting to locate on a diagram a tiny lesion that one cannot see or feel in a breast and that is not in the same position on the operating table that it was when the mammograms were made. There is a slight problem as a result of magnification, and this has been compounded by the recently introduced compression techniques, but with a little experience this causes minimal difficulty.

Biopsy of Occult Breast Carcinoma

CONDICT MOORE, M.D.

Biopsying a lesion that one cannot feel in the human female breast presents the surgeon with a series of interesting technical problems. It is the intention of this paper to present an outline of the way we have attempted to solve these problems. The solutions are not unique or original, but they have worked well in our institution.

First of all, let us define an occult lesion simply as one represented by a suspicious area on a mammogram, one that the examining physician cannot feel, and one that occurs in a patient with no other symptoms that suggest cancer.

There are several rules of thumb we have found useful. The first is to remove a large amount of breast tissue. As a matter of fact, this is advisable even with some palpable lesions, because it is easy to lose a small lesion in the breast once you have incised the skin. The tissue feels and looks different and orientation is quickly lost. To avoid this pitfall, we have developed the standard of taking large biopsies for small lesions. Taking a large piece of tissue provides a wide margin and assures that the lesion is removed the first time. The slight loss of breast volume entailed is far preferable to the mutilation of the breast produced by multiple incisions and reincisions.

The excised piece is a wedge-shaped segment of a breast quadrant. There are three reasons for selecting this shape. First, a better reconstruction can be done. Second, it is easier to carry the incisions down to the fascia overlying the pectoralis major muscle, so that lesions that lie deep in the breast are encompassed by the specimen. Third, the wedge-shaped segment includes the major and the minor ducts and the lobules of breast tissue feeding those ducts. It is a more anatomic and physiologic excision than a slice along one edge or a piece out of the middle.

One little trick that I learned many years ago is to put a single-pronged tenaculum into the breast tissue to be excised. This gives control and does not destroy or compress tissue. It can be used for traction and aids in the orientation of the breast.

Our second rule of thumb is to study the mammograms with the radiologist and the pathologist ahead of time and to determine exactly where the occult lesion lies. Even if we were using diagrams or some other method of localization, I would consider this preoperative study essential.

A third rule of thumb is to perform specimen radiography immediately after excision of the specimen. The preoperative mammograms are, of course, in the operating room for guidance during the biopsy. The surgeon takes these and the specimen to the department of radiology. I think it is worthwhile to take this time to discuss the matter and to make sure that the radiologist promptly supervises specimen radiography. If possible, the pathologist should be there also, so that all three can communicate. If the surgeon waits in the operating room, the others may not feel the immediacy of the situation and a lot of time may be wasted.

We have found it helpful to indicate on the operating schedule that specimen radiography will be needed, just as we list frozen section. We do not, in our system, insist on frozen sections on these very tiny lesions. It also helps to discuss the situation the day before with the radiologist and the pathologist. Since the extra length of anesthesia depends on the time consumed by the specimen radiography, it is important to enlist the cooperation of everyone who will be concerned with the procedure.

Once the specimen has been x-rayed, the film is compared with the preoperative mammograms by the surgeon, the pathologist, and the radiologist in consultation.

The reason for all of this radiographing of the specimen and interdepartmental consultation, as I see it, is to avoid the tragic situation where a lesion is cancer, and the surgeon fails to remove it in his biopsy. This may be because it is too small to see or because the surgeon loses it after incising the skin. The pathologist returns a benign report. The patient is reassured that she does not have cancer. The tumor then grows to palpable size and metastasizes while everybody is resting happily under the false assurance that no cancer can possibly be present. A curable tumor can progress to an incurable one if this happens. Another compelling reason for specimen radiography these days is the need for legal proof of removal of the lesion. This is particularly important in this time of peer review and increased medicolegal activity.

To follow our procedure further, once everyone is assured that the lesion has been removed, the pathologist takes charge of the specimen. Our preference is to close the wound at this point. We prefer not to depend on frozen section for the diagnosis of occult lesions. The patient has been prepared for the performance of biopsy only, for a two-day delay in receiving a final diagnosis, and for the fact that further surgery may be necessary depending on the final diagnosis. This does not mean that the pathologist must not do a frozen section. That is his choice. He can do it if he desires. There will be instances where frozen section will provide an unequivocal, clearcut diagnosis and you can go ahead and make the decision. In general, however, we think it is better to wait for permanent sections in these often tricky diagnostic situations. The patient may have to undergo a second anesthesia, but we feel the risk is less than that of an erroneous frozen section diagnosis. Another benefit of this plan is that the patient can have more participation in the therapeutic decision if she so desires.

The biopsy wound is closed carefully with interrupted catgut, taking care not to strangulate the fatty tissue. Hemostasis must be meticulous. We usually carry out the second procedure, if necessary, in two days.

There is a convenient little technique that our pathologist has developed to help identify the part of the specimen to be sectioned. After taking the specimen radiograph, the film is placed exactly over the specimen, which has not been disturbed. When it has been arranged so that the outlines correspond exactly, a needle is placed through the calcifications on the film into the specimen below, and then the film is taken off of the needle. The tip of the needle then indicates the precise site of the lesion.

We have presented a brief account of how we approach the biopsy of the occult lesion. The whole process takes about 45 minutes because our departments of pathology and radiology are on the same floor and adjacent. We do not wait for frozen section reports. The procedure takes as long as 45 minutes because the surgeon scrubs out and goes to the department of radiology himself. We realize that every surgeon must make individual plans for this occult lesion matter on the basis of the facilities and relationships in his own institution. This plan has worked well for us.

The Pros and Cons of Routine Specimen Radiography

DONALD E. BAUERMEISTER, M.D.

S pecimen radiography is the utilization of radiographic techniques in conjunction with the gross examination of breast biopsy specimens. A question asked frequently is "Should the practicing pathologist in a community hospital setting perform specimen radiography on all breast biopsy material?" In order to answer this question in a complete and logical fashion, one must consider three major issues. First, how cumbersome and time consuming is the technique? Second, what is the yield of occult carcinoma detection by the technique? Third, what alternatives are there if routine specimen radiography is not utilized?

X-ray examination of biopsy material may be accomplished either by using conventional x-ray equipment in a radiology department or by the use of available compact portable industrial instruments such as the Faxitron 805, which can be kept and used in the surgical pathology laboratory. Although adequate images may be obtained in either fashion, the use of the portable equipment is preferred, since its ready accessibility and ease of operation greatly enhance the efficiency of the procedure. Even with this equipment, however, routine specimen radiography is time consuming. To minimize the time involved, we have developed the following procedure. At the time of breast biopsy, if the routine frozen section reveals the lesion to be apparently benign, this report is forwarded to the operating surgeon and the procedure is terminated. Later that day, however, the radiology technician performs specimen radiography on all of the tissue removed, including that utilized for the frozen section. Because of the ease of operation of the Faxitron 805, laboratory personnel can also be trained in its operation.

During the routine gross examination of all surgical pathology material, the pathologist examines the specimen radiograph for the presence of clustered microcalcifications. If such calcifications are found, additional specimen radiographs must be taken in order to localize the lesion. The tissue containing the calcifications is then embedded and separately marked so that serial sections may be taken from this area. It is important to emphasize that in any sections taken of occult calcified lesions, the pathologist must observe the calcifications in the histologic sections before rendering a definitive diagnosis.

It has been our experience and that of others that when specimen radiography is performed in this fashion in patients who have not had the benefit of preoperative mammography, clustered calcifications will be demonstrated in approximately 20% of the biopsy material. This means, therefore, that localizing specimen radiographs must be taken at the time of gross examination and special sections made in approximately one out of every five breast biopsies examined. This may well increase significantly the amount of time spent by the pathologist in his gross examination of breast biopsy material.

Any decision made to initiate this procedure would depend on the answer to our second question, and that is what is the yield of occult carcinoma when this routine is followed? Snyder and Rosen's study, the largest experience yet available, demonstrated that of 4344 initially benign biopsy specimens, significant calcifications were seen in 22%. When these 956 biopsy specimens were radiographically examined, a total of 27 occult carcinomas were detected. This represents an overall yield of occult carcinomas of 0.6%, found by utilizing this technique in a routine fashion. What does this mean to the average practicing pathologist? In most community hospitals, fewer than 200 breast biopsy specimens are processed each year. With this rate of yield, routine specimen radiography could be expected to produce only one additional occult carcinoma per year in these institutions. Considering the time and effort spent, such a low yield would appear to indicate that routine specimen radiography is scarcely practical in the community hospital setting.

What alternatives are available? The answer to this question is that the increasing use of mammography will select those patients in whom clustered microcalcifications are indeed present, and it is in these cases that the usefulness of specimen radiography becomes apparent. In fact, when breast biopsies are performed primarily because of the presence of suspicious microcalcifications not associated with palpable lesions, in other words, mammographically suspicious but clinically occult lesions, specimen radiography is absolutely mandatory. Since this procedure is performed at the time of frozen section and while the patient is under anesthesia, rapid and efficient techniques are essential.

This is a select group of patients, and efficient operation requires them to be flagged in some fashion. This can easily be accomplished if the surgeon schedules the patient for "breast biopsy with specimen radiography." It is advantageous for the pathologist to review the mammogram report prior to the biopsy to acquaint himself with the problem at hand and to be sure that the specimen radiography is indicated. In our institution, it is routine to have preoperative mammograms forwarded to the operating room for all patients who are to undergo biopsy. When the biopsy specimen is brought to the surgical pathology laboratory, the mammograms are delivered simultaneously. A specimen radiograph is made immediately, prior to any dissection of the specimen. With the Faxitron unit, this takes a maximum of one to two minutes. While the films are being developed, the radiologist is notified that his services will be needed in the next few minutes. The pathologist then performs his routine gross examination of the biopsy material by making serial sections approximately 0.5 cm in thickness. If an obvious small carcinoma is encountered, frozen section may be immediately done. If, however, as usually is the case, no gross lesion is seen, the specimen radiograph should be ready for interpretation by the radiologist about the time that the gross examination is completed. If clustered microcalcifications are not seen in the specimen radiographs, the surgeon is advised that additional tissue must be taken. If the calcific lesion has been included in the biopsy specimen, the surgeon is told that the suspicious lesion has been removed and that he may close his incision.

To this point, there has been no delay of the operative procedure beyond that which would have been incurred by routine frozen section. While the surgeon is closing the biopsy incision, a second specimen radiograph is made of the thin slices of breast tissue. This allows accurate localization of the suspicious calcified lesions for subsequent histologic examination. Many centers do not attempt to perform frozen section on this material, since they consider that the undue prolongation in operating time contraindicates this procedure. We have found, however, that we are able to perform the second specimen radiograph and begin frozen section by the time the surgeon has finished closing the biopsy incision. Surgeons are willing to wait an extra five minutes while the frozen section is completed.

On the basis of frozen section, one of three possible reports can be made. If the lesion is clearly malignant, definitive surgical resection may be undertaken immediately. Often, however, small occult lesions are difficult to demonstrate histologically, and even when they are present, the changes are difficult to interpret by frozen section. In this situation, the surgeon is advised of the problem, the procedure is terminated and the final diagnosis is made the following day after examination of permanent sections. If the lesion appears completely benign by frozen section, serial sections may demonstrate foci of occult carcinoma. Therefore the surgeon should delay reassuring the patient until the final surgical pathology report is available.

Finally, what kind of results can be expected when specimen radiography is utilized in conjunction with preoperative mammography? In an attempt to answer this question, we studied 400 consecutive breast biopsies with specimen radiographic techniques. Approximately 90% of the patients had had preoperative mammograms. Fifty-four of the 400 biopsies, or 13.5%, were performed solely because of the presence of clustered microcalcifications demonstrated mammographically. Of these, most turned out to be benign, but 14 clinically occult carcinomas were demonstrated. Seven of these were of microscopic size and undetectable by gross examination. The overall yield of occult carcinomas, therefore, was 3.5%, a sevenfold increase over the detection rate by routine specimen radiography reported by Snyder and Rosen. Applying these statistics, a practicing pathologist in a community hospital who sees 200 breast biopsies a year could expect to find by this technique 7 occult, potentially curable, carcinomas which might otherwise go undetected and therefore untreated. Others have reported even higher detection rates of occult carcinoma with the use of specimen radiography in conjunction with preoperative mammography.

It appears obvious, therefore, that specimen radiography has its greatest utility when used in conjunction with preoperative mammography. In this situation, the use of the technique is mandatory in order to verify that the surgeon has removed the suspicious lesion and to assure that it is thoroughly examined histologically. In institutions where preoperative mammography is not yet utilized to any degree, truly routine specimen radiography appears to be applicable only to a select group of patients. Such patients include those with strong family histories of breast carcinoma, those in whom carcinoma has been demonstrated in the opposite breast, those who have contralateral biopsies performed at the time of mastectomy, and also those patients in whom routine sections have demonstrated significant atypical epithelial hyperplasia. Snyder and Rosen have suggested that radiographic techniques may also be of help in the examination of large breast specimens, in which the sampling error is significant.

Specimen radiography is a mandatory adjunct to mammography if the latter is to be an effective aid in the detection and adequate surgical treatment of early breast carcinoma. Any pathologist who is practicing in an institution in which clinically occult but mammographically suspicious breast lesions are being biopsied and who is not performing specimen radiography is not fulfilling his responsibility to either the surgeon or the patient.

PART FIVE

NEW PROBLEMS
AND NEW SOLUTIONS

What Is a Premalignant Lesion?

ROBERT V. P. HUTTER, M.D.

Thermography and x-ray mammography have increased the yield of nonpalpable, clinically inapparent breast cancers. We in the laboratory are finding ourselves more frequently concerned with purely microscopic, grossly undetectable occult cancers, most of which are noninvasive. The trend, of course, is to find earlier and earlier stages in the evolution of the process. The ultimate intellectual reward of the pseudointellectual pathologist is to be able to diagnose the earliest of the early, before anyone else. So now we are seeking the premalignant lesion.

The definition of premalignant is "preceding the development of malignant characteristics." MacMahon, Hammond, Anderson, Leis, and others have written much about what we call the "premalignant" lesion. In the broadest context, we must regard the female breast as a premalignant target organ when exposed to the physiological milieu of the female organism. While 33,000 women will die of breast cancer this year, only 250 men will succumb to this disease. It is a premalignant condition for a female to live in North America or northern Europe, since the breast cancer rate in these areas is five to six times greater than it is in Asia or Africa. Increasing age is a premalignant condition, since three-fourths of breast cancers occur in women over 40 years of age. A cancer in one breast is a premalignant condition for the opposite breast, since in this country women who have had one breast cancer have at least a five times greater chance of developing cancer in the second breast than women who have not had breast cancer.

A family history of breast cancer is a premalignant condition. In some familial aggregates, as many as 50% of the females develop breast cancer. A woman whose mother or sister has had breast cancer has a two to three times greater risk. If the affected relative had bilateral cancer at an early age, the risk is six to nine times greater and represents a 45% lifetime risk. Daughters of breast cancer patients tend to have their breast cancers at a younger age than their mothers did.

Cyclic ovarian activity, reflected by menarche, pregnancy, and menopause, can be a premalignant condition. The longer the cyclic activity, the greater the risk of breast cancer. It follows that an extended period of cyclic activity is a precancerous condition. Women with menarche before age 16 have a risk of developing breast cancer twice that of those with later menarche. Those with natural menopause after age 55 have twice the risk of those with menopause prior to age 45. Early menopause has the converse effect, decreasing the risk and altering or modifying the premalignant condition. Surgical menopause prior to age 35 reduces the risk by 70% and even prior to age 45 results in a 50% reduction.

Late parity is a premalignant condition. The older the age at the time of the first term delivery, the greater the risk for breast cancer. Women whose first delivery occurs after age 35 have three times the risk of those who deliver before age 18. Although in general, nulliparous women have a higher rate of breast cancer, women who have their first child after age 30 have a greater risk for breast cancer than nulliparous women.

Ovarian and adrenal steroid metabolism may reflect a precancerous state. The work of Bulbrook has indicated that there is a drop in androgen levels prior to the onset of breast cancer. Women who excrete less than 0.4 mg of etiocholanolone in 24 hours have six times the risk of those who excrete more than 1.0 mg. The estrogen profile of Lemon has indicated an increased risk of breast cancer in women in whom the urinary ratio estriol/estradiol + estrone is low.

Women who are obese and have a high fat diet have an increased risk of breast cancer, as do those in the upper socioeconomic strata.

Cancer in certain other organs may represent a premalignant state for primary breast cancer, and vice versa. Patients who have had endometrial carcinoma have twice the risk of developing breast cancer. Patients with ovarian or colon cancer have an increased risk for developing primary breast cancer.

Now, reconsidering that premalignant means the "state preceding the development of malignant characteristics," all of the conditions noted may be considered evidence of a premalignant condition that can be obtained by noninvasive means from the total population of women at risk simply by asking the right questions.

The 90,000 cancers to be diagnosed in 1975 will represent about 20 to 30% of the 100,000 or so breast operations that will be done. Since there are approximately 40,000,000 women at risk, this means that of the 1% of the risk group who have surgery, one of every four will have cancer and we will have tissue from the remaining 0.75% of the total to study for clues of premalignancy.

When we study the tissues from this limited sampling of patients, the recognition of noninvasive or in situ carcinoma is easy, and quite a different problem. The cells of in situ carcinoma are identical to those of invasive carcinoma but have not yet extended beyond their natural habitat. These same cells, once beyond the basement membrane, represent potentially lethal cancer. If in situ carcinoma could be considered the premalignant condition, the task would be greatly simplified. Unfortunately, what we really want is a lesion which is morphologically different from in situ cancer, but which has a great likelihood of becoming in situ and then invasive cancer.

Gallager and Martin have proposed the concept that hyperplasia is a precursor to carcinoma. Let me describe the entire process of cancerous transformation with a quotation: "The more purely cellular hyperplasias may be traced through a series of progressive developments in which changes in the character of the cells are at last apparent. No line of demarcation between the various stages can be made out; they merge insensibly with each other until at last the ducts and acini are filled with cells indistinguishable histologically from cancer cells—intraductal carcinoma. These finally break through the duct wall and invade the tissues forming a cancerous tumor." This description was written by Charteris in the *Journal of Pathology and Bacteriology* in 1930, almost half a century ago.

Chronic cystic mastitis, a benign clinicopathologic entity which represents an exaggeration of the physiologic cyclic activity of the breast, has been considered precancerous. It has three morphologic components: stromal fibrosis, gross or microscopic cysts, and most important, epithelial hyperplasia, which may be diffuse or papillary. Some reports actually include in situ carcinoma as an epithelial element in chronic cystic mastitis, while others do not. The reason for such great variation in the reported incidence of invasive carcinoma in follow-up studies of patients with chronic cystic mastitis is immediately apparent.

There have been numerous studies of the relation of chronic cystic mastitis to carcinoma, many of which were reviewed by Davis, Simons, and Davis in 1964, when they reported the follow-up of their own 284 patients. Seven, or 2.4%, of their patients with cystic mastitis later developed invasive carcinoma. This was 1.7 times the expected rate. In their review of the world literature, the cancer rate was 2.6 times the expected. This is a risk rate based on morphology, comparable to those described earlier which were identified by taking a proper history from the patient.

These authors also recognized the significance of epithelial hyperplasia. In their own patients, those with epithelial hyperplasia (and this included in situ carcinoma) had a rate of invasive cancer 2.5 times the expected, whereas those without epithelial hyperplasia had a rate only 1.2 times the expected. However, and this must be emphasized, almost half of the patients who later developed invasive cancer did so in the breast contralateral to the one originally biopsied.

Various morphologic lesions are included in the category of cystic mastitis and they have been individually studied. Kern and Brooks compared cancerous with noncancerous breasts by studying randomized sections from each. They concluded that cysts were equally as common in cancerous as in noncancerous breasts. Other lesions such as sclerosing adenosis, lobular hyperplasia, and apocrine metaplasia were more common in benign breasts. Atypical and borderline ductal hyperplasia, however, were more common in cancerous breasts.

Black did a retrospective study on patients who had benign biopsies and found the only lesion of precancerous significance was cytologic atypia. Moderate to severe cytologic atypia, not including in situ carcinoma, was associated with five times greater risk for invasive cancer. Black has combined these cases of moderate and severe cytologic atypia with in situ carcinoma and he regards the entire group as precancerous mastopathy. He also found that when patients with precancerous mastopathy developed invasive cancers, the cancers were detected at a more favorable clinical stage, and that the survival characteristics were more favorable than those of cancer patients who had previous benign lesions with no atypia (or prior contralateral invasive cancers).

Silverberg studied noncancerous areas of cancerous breasts and found as other similar studies have shown, a 30% incidence of fibrocystic disease. However, the women with fibrocystic disease and cancer had smaller primary cancers, fewer axillary nodal metastases, and fewer deaths at five years than those who had cancer but no associated fibrocystic disease.

These last two studies suggest that precancerous hyperplasia may stimulate the defense mechanisms of the host to protect against invasive cancer. This, of course, must be taken into account when the choice of therapy is being considered. And, when considering therapy for precancerous mastopathy, it is important to remember that the lesion may be precancerous for either breast.

Before this approach can achieve clinical usefulness, there are several questions that require realistic answers. How much of the breast cancer problem can be accounted for by this type of lesion? If the lesion were fully identified, what should be done about it in an individual patient? MacMahon reports that these precancerous morphologic lesions can account for only about 5% of breast cancers on a population based study. Thus the most we could expect, if we were completely successful with the microscope, is the prevention of about 5000 cancers per year. I do not belittle this, but it is obvious that we need to do more to reach the other 95% of women destined to develop clinical breast cancer. This must be done by taking all factors into account, properly weighing them by multifactorial regression analysis and devising a modular decision system for action.

In closing, I would like to caution against the hazards of success in the identification and ablation of premalignant lesions. Success will eventually evoke what I refer to as the phenomenon of alternating generations of physicians. Having achieved our objective, no more patients will develop metastases or die from breast cancer. Under present conditions the fact that patients continue to die is our security blanket, our assurance that the lesions we have identified are really cancer. When the next generation comes along and there are no deaths, they will challenge us for calling these lesions precancerous since, after all, no one ever gets breast cancer.

The Management of Premalignant or Histologically Dubious Lesions: A Panel Discussion

MODERATOR: JOHN E. MARTIN, M.D.
CHARLES W. HAYDEN, M.D.
WILLIAM E. POWERS, M.D.
WILLIAM W. SHINGLETON, M.D.
REUVEN K. SNYDERMAN, M.D.
HERBERT B. TAYLOR, M.D.

DR. MARTIN: Tell me, Dr. Taylor, what do you consider to be a borderline lesion?

DR. TAYLOR: One definition that I like is that a borderline lesion is one that somebody else calls cancer and I call benign. Or we could say that borderline lesions are those about which a panel of experts could not agree.

DR. MARTIN: Do you think in situ carcinoma is a precursor to invasive cancer?

DR. TAYLOR: Yes. Fred Stewart used to say about carcinoma in situ of the cervix "If the invasive cancer does not come from in situ cancer, where does it come from?" I think the same thing is true in the breast.

DR. MARTIN: That is fair enough. Do you think intraductal carcinoma is clinically significant? How long is it going to be before it invades?

DR. TAYLOR: That depends on how long it has been there, of course. If we use the standard epidemiological approach, and the average age of women with intraductal carcinoma is 10 years less than that of those with invasion, we can say it takes 10 years before intraductal cancer becomes invasive cancer. But when you see a patient with intraductal cancer, you do not know how long it has been there. It may have been there nine and a half years. She may have used all the lead time. The epidemiologists have proved that there are quantitative considerations as well as qualitative. A patient with a lot of in situ cancer is probably closer to invasion than one with a little bit.

DR. MARTIN: Dr. Hayden, Dr. Shingleton, how do you treat these noninvasive cancers?

DR. HAYDEN: I have gone pretty much full circle. When I started doing operations for in situ carcinoma, I did local excisions. A lot of those patients are still alive. Then, however, I began to encounter patients who had in situ carcinoma in one quadrant and invasion in another, and I went back to my original Halstedian principles and did radical mastectomies. Subsequently, I backed off to modified radical mastectomy and now I am doing total mastectomy and taking out a few nodes. For the atypias, I have been using quadrant excisions and close follow-up with physical examinations and mammography. The second breast is an entirely different problem. If there were a carcinoma in one breast and I found an area of atypia in the second, I would recommend selective prophylactic total mastectomy.

DR. SHINGLETON: That certainly reflects my own thinking. The most important thing is to keep an open mind. Information is lacking upon which to make good decisions at the present time. I, by nature, tend to be conservative. For example, for carcinoma in situ, I would consider partial mastectomy, or at most simple mastectomy. The question about multicentricity is critical, in my opinion. Until we get more information about that I am not sure that our selection of operations can be too rational.

DR. MARTIN: How do you differentiate lumpectomy from partial mastectomy?

DR. SHINGLETON: Lumpectomy is a vague term. It can mean just an excision of a mass with a little surrounding breast tissue, or it can mean removal of one-fourth of the breast.

DR. MARTIN: Dr. Powers, what if one of these surgeons did a lumpectomy on a patient with severe atypia? What would you do with that breast?

DR. POWERS: Probably nothing. We are caught between our interest in saving this woman's breast and saving her life. The upsurge of interest in breast cancer is going to make life a lot more difficult for pathologists and surgeons in making decisions on earlier and earlier cases. The fact is, that with one of these diagnoses of probable cancer, we have to take some risk. Already we are taking risks in such ways as doing axillary dissections for a small proportion of probably positive nodes and for an even smaller proportion of people with positive nodes who can be cured. In these early or dubious carcinomas, one can get a very high cure rate. The only problem is that you sacrifice the woman's breast. I hope the day will come when lumpectomy will be used not only in Stage 1 breast cancer, but also in this situation. At present, however, I am not prepared to do it.

It can be argued that one of the problems of treating a patient with an invasive breast cancer with radiation is that there may be late carcinogenesis. I would argue that the probability of carcinoma developing in the opposite breast is far greater than that of carcinoma in the breast that has been treated. If, however, there were a group of patients in whom I could see good reason for concern about carcinoma being engendered by radiation, it might be these patients with borderline lesions. To treat them by radiation would be to subject them to a carcinogenic agent, and this in patients in whom the cure rate by alternative means might be tremendously high.

DR. MARTIN: Dr. Shingleton and Dr. Hayden, what do you think about lobular carcinoma in situ? How do you handle these cases?

DR. HAYDEN: Lobular carcinoma in situ is an at risk cancer and should be treated by the removal of the breast.

DR. MARTIN: An opposite breast biopsy?

DR. HAYDEN: Yes, especially in younger individuals. I have also done bilateral total mastectomy occasionally and referred the patient for reconstruction. I have personally had the experience of having what seemed to be a pure carcinoma in situ only to find that there were one or two positive nodes from a tiny focus of invasive carcinoma in that breast.

DR. SHINGLETON: I feel that for lobular carcinoma in situ, total mastectomy with a biopsy of the opposite breast is indicated. If no lesion were found in the second breast, I would encourage the patient to get repeated mammograms at least once a year. I do not favor doing a bilateral total mastectomy under these circumstances.

DR. MARTIN: Dr. Taylor, does the infrequency of recurrence with these in situ carcinomas have anything to do with the time lag in the development of lesions?

DR. TAYLOR: I think it could very well. Most of the reports describing the results of subtotal mastectomy are of relatively recent origin, and it may be that the latent interval is such that there has not been a chance for development of these multicentric foci into clinical cancer.

DR. MARTIN: Dr. Shingleton, how can we educate surgeons to do a generous biopsy when they cannot palpate a lesion? Can you start an education program for surgeons?

DR. SHINGLETON: I think one has been started. I am not sure how effective it has been up to the present, but at least in our medical school we are trying to get the message across. A large percentage of the surgery done for carcinoma of the breast is actually done in small community hospitals. The Cancer Control Program of the National Cancer Institute is specifically designed to disseminate information to community hospitals and to the surgeons, pathologists, and radiologists who work in them so that they can appreciate the developments which are in progress.

DR. POWERS: I am impressed that, in a practical sense, much of the education is coming from diagnostic radiologists. They are pushing surgeons to find these lesions that are found on mammograms. There is one problem that has been bothering me, and I would like some help with it. Often a report of a mammogram comes to a surgeon saying so-and-so has been found and "biopsy is advised." Many surgeons are reluctant to do a biopsy just because a radiologist has suggested it. Is that the proper wording to put in the report? Or, should one say "biopsy should be considered"? Then that gives the surgeon the opportunity of thinking about it and discussing it with the patient and with the radiologist.

DR. MARTIN: I think that is a matter between individual radiologists and surgeons. I tend to report in histologic terms, but if I do not know the referring physician very well, I will specifically say that a suspect focus should be biopsied because I think this is my prerogative and duty as a consultant.

DR. SHINGLETON: Is there a medicolegal aspect to this?

DR. MARTIN: I really do not know. In a way I do not see much difference between this situation and one in which the surgeon feels a mass and tells the patient a biopsy is necessary.

DR. SHINGLETON: It is the same general situation.

DR. MARTIN: Dr. Snyderman, we have been leaving you over there to ruminate on all these thoughts. In these patients with so-called premalignant or minimal lesions, or minimally invasive lesions, would you recommend subcutaneous mastectomy and prosthesis? Suppose a biopsy showed atypical duct hyperplasia?

DR. SNYDERMAN: If the report were available ahead of time, no. I would not recommend the use of subcutaneous mastectomy for either severe atypia or in situ carcinoma. There is another point though. If the total mastectomy is done preserving the muscle, without use of a skin graft and without post-operative therapy, a fairly pleasant reconstruction can be accomplished if it is desired. The difference between these two procedures in terms of the result of reconstruction is not that great.

DR. MARTIN: Do you do mammograms on patients who have augmentations?

DR. SNYDERMAN: Every breast operation I do is preceded by a mammogram.

DR. HAYDEN: Does the presence of a prosthesis interfere with interpretation? Does the radiologist have any difficulty?

DR. SNYDERMAN: Those I have spoken with say they do not. If they want to examine the tissue around the implant they have to use a different type of positioning, but this is no problem.

DR. MARTIN: Do you favor subcutaneous mastectomy in patients who have had multiple biopsies or who have family histories of breast cancer?

DR. SNYDERMAN: If they have had multiple biopsies and are going to have more, I think this is a good indication for the procedure. If there is a family history in addition that is another point in favor of it.

DR. MARTIN: Would you explain why you object to subcutaneous mastectomy for in situ carcinoma?

DR. SNYDERMAN: A subcutaneous mastectomy leaves behind some breast tissue, probably about 5% of the total, especially behind the nipple. In the type of mastectomy that should be done for cancer, the flaps are so thin that you cannot and should not insert a prosthesis immediately. This is necessary in order to be sure that breast tissue is not left behind. The subcutaneous mastectomy with implant gives the patient a feeling of security which she should not have.

DR. MARTIN: I think we will open the discussion to the audience at this point.

QUESTION: In these premalignant lesions and in situ lesions, it has been indicated that there should be careful follow-up with frequent mammograms. Is it possible that these borderline lesions might be stimulated by these small amounts of radiation?

DR. POWERS: I guess there is a hypothetical basis for considering that there would be some possible damage to these patients but I do not think the risk is great. Probably the risk of cancer associated with not doing anything is greater.

QUESTION: This is in response to Dr. Shingleton's question. When I find something that may be cancer but is not completely diagnostic, I sit down and talk to the patient myself and say, "There is something equivocal in your breast, and I am going to recommend that you have a biopsy." I think the patient should be taken into the radiologist's confidence and that the surgeon should not have to bear the brunt of the decision.

DR. SHINGLETON: This is a good point. The patient ought to be involved in decision making.

DR. MARTIN: I'm afraid we've used up all our time. Thank you, gentlemen, and thank you, audience, for your interest.

Reflections on Benign Disease: A Radiographic-Histologic Correlation

JOHN E. MARTIN, M.D.
H. STEPHEN GALLAGER, M.D.

Mammography heretofore has been concerned largely with the recognition of patterns diagnostic of carcinoma. Abnormalities representing nonneoplastic and benign processes have been characterized only to the extent necessary to differentiate them from malignant disease. There is a tendency to attribute all such changes to the vaguely defined entity, fibrocystic disease, and to pay little attention to the specific histologic changes responsible. This lack of precision is compounded by the general inconsistency of the histopathologic terminology applied to benign breast lesions. This paper reports the results of an attempt to resolve this problem by making specific correlations between certain benign mammographic appearances and their histologic counterparts.

A series of 50 patients was studied. All exhibited mammographic changes of benign disease and all had biopsies. Multiple sections from each biopsy specimen were reviewed. The histologic lesions present in each patient were recorded in accordance with a predetermined categorization system (Table 1). Similarly, all mammographic abnormalities were recorded. In each case, a predominant type of lesion was indicated. Although point-for-point correlation was not possible because of the random orientation and incomplete sampling provided by the biopsy sections, some statistical validity has been achieved by the number of examples included.

The common benign lesions of the breast were found to fall into three

Table 1   Histologic Lesions Recorded

Lobular hyperplasia	Duct ectasia
Florid adenosis	Fat necrosis
Sclerosing adenosis	Fibroadenoma
Inappropriate persistence of lobules	Fibroadenomatoid mastopathy
Inappropriate lobular activity	Indurative mastopathy
Papillary duct hyperplasia	Galactocele
Nonpapillary duct hyperplasia	Duct hyperplasia with atypia
Cyst (epithelial)	Lobular hyperplasia with atypia
Cyst (nonepithelial)	Noninvasive lobular carcinoma
Abscess	Noninvasive ductal carcinoma

broad categories: (a) those due to variations in normal structure, (b) those due to one or another of the manifestations of epithelial hyperplasia, and (c) those resulting from periductal mastitis. In some individuals all three causative factors were operative simultaneously.

The normal breast contains 15 to 25 major duct systems radiating outward from the nipple. In the nipple and subareolar region, the major ducts have diameters of 0.5 to 0.8 mm. Branching begins about a centimeter below the base of the nipple, or at the edge of the areola in the case of ducts that are directed more laterally, and proceeds in a complex fashion into the peripheral portions of the breast. Each duct in the young female terminates in one or several clusters of coiled ductules called lobules. Lobules are few in the nipple, subareolar region, and central portion of the breast, but numerous in the periphery. In most patients there are a few fine, short, twiglike branches arising from major ducts in the central region and an occasional individual has a large amount of lobular tissue in the nipple and subareolar region.

With each menstrual cycle, some of the lobules undergo enlargement. These, if pregnancy does not supervene, subsequently atrophy completely leaving blind ending ducts. At any time during menstrual life, therefore, the breast contains inactive lobules, lobules in process of enlarging, and those in various stages of atrophy. The number of lobules in a single breast is not constant through life, but decreases progressively with each menstrual cycle. The rate of lobular regression accelerates at menopause.

Around and between the ducts and lobules in the active breast is a mass of sparsely cellular collagenous connective tissue. That immediately surrounding the ducts tends, at least in young women, to stain more intensely with eosin than that more distant from ducts. This observation leads to the suspicion, as yet unconfirmed, that there are two types of stroma in the normal breast, possibly of differing cellular origin. Throughout menstrual life, there is a gradual loss of this collagenous background tissue, more or less paralleling the reduction in number of lobules. As the dense stroma diminishes, it is replaced by adipose tissue. There are several known factors that increase the rate and extent of this fatty replacement, including lactation, obesity, a diet high in carbohydrate, and acute systemic disease.

The basic lesion of the fibrocystic disease complex is hyperplasia of mammary epithelium, either ductal or lobular or both. It is regularly accompanied by an increase in stromal connective tissue, probably of the periductal variety. As the number of cells in a duct increases, the duct elongates, becomes tortuous, and folds upon itself. Points of sharp angulation of the wall become necrotic, the lining epithelium loses its ability to reproduce, and a cyst is thus formed. Ultimately, the epithelium lining the cyst may undergo complete atrophy. Under these circumstances, the cyst content, consisting as it does of the detritus of epithelial destruction and the degeneration products of blood, is apparently sufficiently irritating to produce a mild local inflammatory reaction. While the duct cells are increasing in fibrocystic disease, lobules also may increase focally in both size and number as a result of an increase in the number of their component cells.

All of the various components in this complex process are usually present in every involved breast, but not necessarily to the same degree. Duct hyperplasia and cyst formation may predominate in one specimen, fibrosis in another. The numerous combinations of lesions possible accounts for the bewildering variety of clinical presentations included under the general heading of fibrocystic disease.

Periductal mastitis, by contrast, is an inflammatory disease affecting the larger mammary ducts. Its etiology is unknown, but it is suspected that the disease is related to poor nipple hygiene. Early in this prolonged and indolent process, there is ulceration of the epithelium of one or more of the large central ducts. The surrounding connective tissue becomes filled with a mixture of inflammatory cells, producing the histologic picture of plasma cell mastitis. Exudative fluid fills the lumina of the involved ducts. In the healing phase, periductal fibrosis becomes prominent, and the rigid walled ducts assume calibers greater than normal (duct ectasia). The fluid within the ducts may resorb, or it may organize by coagulation and ingrowth of fibroblasts from the ulcerated duct wall. Subsequently, regeneration of epithelium from intact portions of the duct may occur with the production of fibrotic pseudopapillomata.

Normal anatomic structures are reflected in all mammograms. The ducts of largest diameter in the subareolar area are usually visible, but smaller ducts are beyond the resolving power of the procedure, as are also lobules of normal size. Bilaterally symmetrical, uniformly dilated ducts in the subareolar regions are probably a normal variant related to cyclic breast activity. The uniform density that characterizes the young or active breast is the mammographic image of the dense collagenous stroma normal at this age, and does not indicate the presence of disease.

In mammograms, ducts in the nipple and subareolar region often are seen to be dilated. When the enlarged ducts are multiple and symmetrical, the most frequent cause is periductal mastitis. The enlargement is due both to the increase in duct caliber and to the ensheathing layer of reactive fibrous tissue. A similar appearance in older patients is often simply the result of progressive involution of the breast.

The presence of unilateral dilated subareolar ducts, especially when solitary or few in number, is a more ominous sign invariably indicative of significant disease. This appearance also may be the result of periductal mastitis, or it may reflect duct papilloma or intraductal carcinoma. If the dilated duct system extends 2 or 3 cm into the breast and has a beaded contour, either a papilloma or the fibrotic pseudopapilloma of periductal mastitis is the usual etiology. The two are indistinguishable mammographically. Isolated dilated ducts of smooth outline also have a variety of causes. Most often they represent the ectatic ducts of late periductal mastitis, but structures of this type may also be found to contain papillomatous lesions of either type. It is to be emphasized that, since true papilloma is a product of epithelial hyperplasia, and since hyperplasia is a nonobligate preneoplastic lesion, concomitant carcinoma must always be considered a distinct possibility.

Cysts may be imaged mammographically in many ways. They are represented more accurately by the xeroradiographic process than by films, chiefly because of the edge enhancement phenomenon and because the higher resolution clarifies the nature of surrounding densities. A solitary cyst with clearly defined borders, particularly one that fluctuates in size with the phases of the menstrual cycle or disappears on subsequent studies, is usually one that histologically has a normal epithelial lining and contains clear fluid. A solitary cyst that remains unchanged, however, is usually found to have flattened, atrophic epithelium or to have lost its lining altogether, and to be filled with opaque, pasty green-brown material.

The lack of a discrete border in the mammographic image of a cyst is a sign that inflammatory changes have occurred, usually as a result of loss of epithelium. The consequent surrounding fibrosis merges in density with the mammary stroma. Such cysts can be made to change in contour by compression, a helpful radiographic sign.

Small cysts (microcysts) usually are lined by epithelium, occur in clusters, and are readily mistaken for small knobby carcinomas. Apocrine metaplasia, an epithelial alteration of no serious significance, may occur in cysts of any size and is not specifically reflected mammographically. An occasional cyst contains large amounts of lipid substance and is therefore more lucent than the background. The reason for this is not yet known.

Adenosis, hyperplasia of mammary lobules, is shown mammographically as a large number of snowflakelike densities, the result of the increase in size and number of the lobules. The minute, diffuse calcifications which may accompany this process are a manifestation of altered metabolism of calcium by the hyperplastic cells. When adenosis is associated with ductal hyperplasia or carcinoma, the related increase in collagenous stroma may obscure the delicate lobular image. Sclerosing adenosis, the regressive form of lobular hyperplasia, also eventuates in the obliteration of the individual images of the enlarged lobular clusters, leaving only the calcifications as an indication of abnormality. The calcifications of adenosis and sclerosing adenosis frequently appear in clusters and are round or semiround and coarse. These calcifications can usually be differentiated from the calcifications of duct carcinoma, which are usually irregular, rodlike, or branching. The calcific clusters associated with adenosis and sclerosing adenosis cannot be differentiated from those of invasive lobular carcinoma or lobular carcinoma in situ. Occasionally, foci of lobular carcinoma in situ are found adjacent to benign lobular calcifications.

Lack of bilateral symmetry in the contour of the mammary tissue has long been recognized as a sign suggestive of carcinoma. When carcinoma is present, assymmetry is the result of the unilateral increase in periductal collagen which accompanies the development of carcinoma. The sign itself, however, is basically the result of a focal increase in stromal connective tissue and may have any of a number of causes or even a combination of causes. Epithelial hyperplasia, for example, may be accompanied by proliferation of collagen-producing connective tissue. Periductal mastitis leads to fibrosis as a result of scarring. Some degree of asymmetry may even be a normal variation. It is not our intent to suggest that asymmetry should be ignored, but only to point out that in many cases, perhaps a majority, it is due to factors other than carcinoma.

The results of this study, while necessarily preliminary and tentative, indicate the possibility of identifying specific benign lesions by their mammographic images. It is planned to continue this work with the hope that it will become possible to identify by mammography lesions that have significant propensities for subsequent development of carcinoma.

Bilateral Breast Cancer:
How Frequent;
How to Find It;
What to Do about It:
A Panel Discussion

Moderator: RICHARD G. LESTER, M.D.
DAVID E. ANDERSON, Ph.D.
ROBERT L. EGAN, M.D.
ROBERT V. P. HUTTER, M.D.
HENRY P. LEIS, JR., M.D.
JEROME A. URBAN, M.D.

DR. LESTER: The subject of this panel is the serious, important, and vexing problem of bilateral breast cancer. There are many issues within this area. What is bilateral breast cancer? What should be done about it? Is this a preventable disease? Under what circumstances should prophylactic therapy be considered?

There is an analogy between breast cancer and lung cancer. Both are probably multicentric in origin, at least in some cases. In the one case, however, we are dealing with an organ that is accessible; in the other, one that is internal. In one case the entire system cannot be surgically ablated. In the other, total ablation is conceivable, if undesirable. We rarely recognize multicentric lung cancer clinically because survivorship is so low. In breast cancer, however, survivals are improving and, consequently, bilaterality is a practical clinical question for us and for our patients. I have asked Dr.

Anderson to start this discussion and to talk about the statistics of the problem, as well as his own work.

DR. ANDERSON: The subject of this session is "new problems and new solutions," and I submit that bilateral breast cancer is not a new problem, although it may require new solutions. Bilaterality has been reported and described for many years. We have heard repeatedly that cancer in one breast is the most frequent precancerous lesion for the other breast. We have also heard repeatedly that cancer in one breast increases the risk of cancer developing in the opposite breast five- to sevenfold.

The reported figures for frequency of bilateral breast cancer are variable. The rate found depends on the type of material that one is working with, the initial stage of disease, the length of the follow-up periods, and so forth. In a series of 6000 patients reported several years ago, we found a frequency of bilaterality of 2.7%. In this study there was no consideration for stage of disease, site, or period of follow-up. Robbins and Berg, using a 20 year follow-up, found a frequency of 6.4%. In another study with a six year follow-up, the rate was 1.9%.

If one resorts to biopsy of the opposite breast, the frequency of bilaterality appears to increase, suggesting that the problem is more frequent than we realize. I suspect that it seems more frequent because some of the tumors found may represent metastatic disease. On the other hand, in the genetic type of breast cancer with which we have been concerned, bilateral primaries are similar histologically. If similar lesions in opposite breasts were all considered metastatic, this would tend to underestimate the frequency of true bilaterality.

There is also the problem of multicentric tumors. If a tumor is multicentric in one breast, it might seem to increase the probability that one in the contralateral breast would be metastatic. I would suggest, however, that bilaterality is just another expression of multiplicity. A person may be predisposed to multiple lesions, and they may develop from multiple developing foci in both breasts.

As I reported earlier, patients who have family histories of breast cancer have a high frequency of bilateral disease. It should be pointed out that there are several neoplasms that seem to have genetic components and also to be frequently multicentric. Classic examples are familial polyposis of the colon and medullary carcinoma of the thyroid. Multicentricity or bilaterality is a characteristic of genetically oriented neoplasms and is by no means unique to breast cancer.

DR. EGAN: Early in my experience I was impressed with the ease with which mammography can differentiate between primary and metastic disease. We can resolve this problem almost at a glance. Another thing that impressed me was the frequency with which we found contralateral tumors by mammography as compared to clinical examination. Haagensen reported bilaterality in only 0.4% of his patients and we were finding a rate of 4% at M. D. Anderson Hospital, a tenfold difference.

Bilateral breast cancer may be simultaneous or nonsimultaneous, metastatic or second primary. Metastatic disease is of importance only as it bears on staging. Frequently, however, second primaries are labeled as metastatic disease. Most cancers in opposite breasts are not metastatic, even in advanced disease. We found in 75 cases that 59 of the cancers in the opposite breast were truly second primaries. The differentiation of second primaries from metastic disease is quite simple. The second primary looks like a primary cancer. The diagnosis in the second breast is made on the same signs as in the first. In metastatic disease, however, the breast is diffusely more dense. No mass is seen. There is indistinctness of structure in this overall density and widespread thickening of the skin.

At Emory University in the last 10 years, we have done 16,000 examinations on 3000 patients and found 82 bilateral cancers. Some developed under observation. Of this group, 65, or 80%, were primaries, and the remainder were metastases. This compares well with the rate reported by Robbins and Berg. Out of 1100 patients followed for 20 years, they found 91 second primaries. Our patients have been followed a shorter time, yet our number of second primaries is almost the same. This emphasizes the help that mammography offers in this problem.

DR. LESTER: If, indeed, we are to have an impact on the problem of bilateral disease, we must know how the pathologist can help us and how early he can help us. Dr. Hutter, will you talk to us about bilaterality from the standpoint of the pathologist?

DR. HUTTER: The only thing that has changed in the last 50 years is that what we pathologists have been saying all along is now being listened to, and I think that we can thank mammography for that. If one looks at the older reports—before the last decade—the figures for bilaterality are much lower than they are now. Why are there such changes? The main reason is that the old reports were based on palpable lumps, clinical cancers. Now we are deriving information from the sort of work that Urban and others are doing, where biopsies are being done on asymptomatic contralateral breasts and microscopic findings are available. The incidence is much higher because we are talking about two different stages of the disease.

It is important to make an assessment as to whether a contralateral lesion represents new primary or metastatic cancer. Obviously the therapeutic implications are profound. Robbins and Berg established criteria for this distinction in their 20 year follow-up study. The most significant factor is the finding of in situ areas in the second breast. Primary cancers occur within the breast substance, in contradistinction to metastases, which come from sub-cutaneous lymphatics or through vascular dissemination and are found in fatty tissue or lymph nodes. The presence of tumor outside of the breast substance itself is a clue that the lesion may be metastatic rather than primary.

The second primary is expansile, usually stellate, and appears as a solitary dominant mass, whereas metastases may be multiple. Second primaries tend to be in a mirror image location. If the first cancer was in the inner lower quadrant of one breast, the second will probably occur in the inner lower quadrant of the other. Forty percent of second primaries are histologically identical to the first primary. The rigid criteria applied before the Robbins and Berg study required that the second cancer be histologically different, but that is nonsense.

I would like to describe some illustrative cases that have a bearing on this problem. The first was a patient who had a 2 cm cancer excised for biopsy, then had a mastectomy. After this specimen was routinely examined and reported out as showing no residual cancer, we did whole organ studies and found 38 areas of carcinoma; 32 in situ, 6 infiltrating. One wonders what the incidence of multicentricity actually is. Another woman who had a localized carcinoma removed had only one area of cancer found by whole organ sectioning. A third woman, who was 80 years old, was hospitalized because of a fracture of the neck of the femur as the result of a fall. She had a large breast cyst, and a mastectomy was performed. In this specimen, we found 3 separate areas of invasive cancer, 54 areas of papillomatosis, 54 areas of atypical hyperplasia, 22 areas of intraductal carcinoma, and 10 scattered areas of focal calcification.

Finally, we studied a group of patients to determine the significance of mammographic findings in patients with known lobular carcinoma in situ. These 61 patients all had lobular carcinoma in situ to begin with and all had clinical mammograms. It turned out, in this highly selected group that there was 65% bilaterality.

Since many of the lesions we are concerned with in determining bilaterality are noninvasive, let me bring out something about the pathologic differentiation between atypia and carcinoma in situ. Atypia is different things not only to different people but to the same person under varying circumstances. We do not interpret the same morphologic evidence in the same way every time. If you were to show me a biopsy from a young woman with some cytologic atypia, and the patient had no family background of cancer and no other alarming factors, I would call that atypia and feel that the patient should have the ordinary type of follow-up. If you showed me an identical lesion from another woman, maybe 55, whose mother, grandmother, three sisters, and daughter have had breast cancer and who herself has had cancer in one breast, I would feel that this should be acted upon. In all honesty, we have to say we are not objective. I think this is the difference between good science and good medicine.

DR. LESTER: Dr. Urban has had considerable experience with elective biopsy of the contralateral breast, and I have asked him to talk to us on this subject.

DR. URBAN: Our interest in this problem was stimulated by a patient we saw in 1958, who had a biopsy of one breast which disclosed a 2 cm infiltrating cancer, but who also had two large nodes in the opposite axilla. It would have been easy to assume that this was metastatic from the palpable tumor. There was no mass in the second breast. We biopsied one node and surveyed the patient thoroughly. There was no evidence of systemic disease. Biopsy showed a 0.6 cm carcinoma in the tail of the contralateral breast which we could not feel and which the pathologist was lucky to find. She has remained free of disease for 16 years.

A few years later, in evaluating the statistical follow-up on the extended radicals, we were amazed to find that 9% of the original patients undergoing extended radical for infiltrating cancer had developed clinically apparent cancers in their opposite breasts. This was 15% of the surviving group. Gradually, with growing awareness of the importance of the second breast, we decided to biopsy opposite breasts routinely in patients with known cancers. In 120 patients with no x-ray or physical signs in their opposite breast, 10% of the biopsies showed carcinoma of the opposite breast. When there were minimal clinical or x-ray signs, biopsies showed carcinoma in almost 18%. Adding it all up, 14% of our biopsies disclosed cancer in the opposite breast. When there was infiltrating cancer in the dominant breast, half of the contralateral carcinomas were infiltrating and half noninfiltrating. When there was noninfiltrating cancer in the first breast, almost all the carcinomas in the other were noninfiltrating. This suggests that the lesions had started to develop at about the same time in both breasts.

In a second series based on clinic material, only 43% of opposite breasts were biopsied, but the bilaterality index was similar—16%. In this group, 10% were sequential and 6% simultaneous. The advantage of this approach is pointed out by the fact that two-thirds of the contralateral cancers were noninfiltrating, and only one of the infiltrating cancers had positive nodes in the axilla. By contrast, in 236 patients who were followed after previous mastectomy and who developed contralateral primaries, only a quarter had noninfiltrating cancer.

There is no really reliable method for detecting early breast cancer. Of the bilateral patients in whom we utilized x-ray mammography, 7 patients had mammograms positive on both sides, 11 were positive on one side, and 12 were negative on both sides. You have to use all methods of diagnosis to maximize detection, and contralateral biopsy is one of these methods.

DR. LESTER: Dr. Leis, will you tell us how you recognize the patient who is at high risk and when you advise prophylactic contralateral mastectomy?

DR. LEIS: The reported incidence of bilateral primary breast cancer of the simultaneous type when based on clinically detectable cancer ranges from 0.2 to 2%, with an average of about 0.5%. However, if one includes preclinical or presymptomatic cancers, less than the clinically palpable size of 1 cm, this figure would probably be over 3%. I have reported an incidence of 0.3% for simultaneous bilateral clinically detectable cancer and of 3.3% for preclinical bilateral cancer detected by mammography in a series of 504 patients who had clinically detectable cancers in the first breasts. Urban's random biopsies of opposite breasts at the time of the initial mastectomy found an incidence rate of 14.3%. One-third of these cancers were infiltrating and two-thirds were not. Critics of this work emphasize that the clinical significance of noninfiltrating cancer is still the subject of considerable controversy and that lobular carcinoma in situ is nonlethal and frequently does not go on to invasive cancer. While this is true, Hutter and Foote in a long term follow-up of patients with lobular carcinoma in situ found that 33% developed invasive cancers.

Most authorities recommend at least subcutaneous or complete simple mastectomy for noninvasive cancers. If such a cancer is found in a second breast, it would seem logical to apply the same treatment that would be selected for the lesion if it were found in the first breast.

In carefully selected patients in whom I have performed prophylactic removal of the second breast, a bilaterality rate similar to that reported by Urban has been obtained. Seventeen unsuspected cancers were found in 97 cases, an incidence of 17.5%. About one-third of these were infiltrating and two-thirds were not.

The reported incidence of nonsimultaneous second primary breast cancer ranges from 1 to 12% with an average of about 7%. Slack, Bross, Nemoto, and Fisher found only 52 cases among 2734 patients from the National Adjuvant Breast Project study from 1961 to 1968, a rate of 1.9%. In contradistinction, Shah, Rosen, and Robbins reported a series from Memorial Hospital in which 110 cases of bilateral breast cancer were found in a total of 508 patients (21.6%).

Certainly the figure of 7% for bilateral breast cancer is not impressive, but it does not reflect the true picture. The combined 5 year survival rate for Stage 1 and Stage 2 breast cancer is only about 60% and the 10 year rate is much lower. Many patients do not live long enough to have much chance of developing cancer in the remaining breast. The incidence of cancer in the second breast increases at the rate of about 1% per year of survival. If only those patients with early cancers and good prognoses for long term survival were considered, the incidence figure would be much higher. The frequency of cancer in the second breast is directly related to the stage of the cancer in the first breast. Many series do not have long term follow-ups, many cases being followed for only five years. The longer the follow-up, the higher the percentage of cancers in the second breast will be. A third variable is whether breast-years or patient-years are considered in the incidence rates. Robbins and Berg estimated that the risk of developing cancer in the second breast is about five times that for the general population. Patients with only one breast have only one-half the risk of the population as a whole, and thus the risk would be doubled if breast-years rather than patient-years were used in reporting. Further, noninvasive cancers have a higher incidence of bilaterality than invasive ones, the highest incidence being in lobular carcinoma in situ, which has a bilaterality rate of 35 to 40%. The incidence of cancer developing in the second breast in patients with early cancers in the first breast, who have good prognoses for long term survival, who have a long term (20 year) follow-up, and whose statistical incidence is based on breast-years rather than patient-years is at least 20 to 30%.

There is a group of patients who are especially prone to develop cancer in the second breast. This "high risk" group includes (a) patients with noninvasive cancers, (b) patients with favorable types of invasive cancer such as colloid, medullary with lymphoid infiltrate, comedo with minimal stromal invasion, and papillary, (c) patients whose first cancer was Stage 1, especially those under 1 cm, (d) patients with family histories of breast cancer, (e) patients with multiple primary cancers in the first breast, (f) patients in whom random biopsy of the second breast shows precancerous mastopathy, and (g) patients who are under 50 years of age at the time of their first cancer.

The breasts are paired organs and should be considered as an anatomic system rather than as separate and unrelated. They are linked by lymphatic and vascular pathways and are under the same genetic and hormonal influences. Removing one breast for cancer certainly does not prevent the carcinogenic factors influential in producing the first lesion from exerting the same influence on the opposite breast.

Much is made of the psychologic and physical importance of the remaining breast after mastectomy. Lewison and Neto feel that it provides psychologic support for many women who cherish it as a badge of motherhood, a sign of feminity, and a psychosexual symbol. Haagensen has written that surgeons who "are humanists as well as scientists, know that her second breast is an important asset for a woman who has lost one breast." The remaining breast, however, is useless and largely nonfunctional. Few women are willing to show it as a badge of sexual enhancement alongside their mastectomy scar and few women allow it to be used during the act of lovemaking. If the patient were to become pregnant and be allowed to deliver, it would be rare indeed that the patient would allow, or the doctor condone, its use for nursing. The remaining breast, especially if it is large, results in loss of symmetry. The patient feels unbalanced and has difficulty in dressing, bathing, and movements. The large breasted woman is often forced to wear a cumbersome and uncomfortable prosthesis at night as well as in the daytime in an attempt to match the other breast.

Patients live in a constant fear that carcinoma will develop in the remaining breast and that another extensive surgical procedure will be necessary with, at best, a questionable cure rate. Their fear is certainly justified, since cancer in the second breast deleteriously influences survival. Robbins and Berg noted that a second breast cancer almost halved the expected survival time.

In management of a cancer in the second breast, it is paramount to determine whether it is primary or metastatic. When it is of a different histologic type than the cancer in the first breast, it is presumed to be a new primary. When the histologic patterns are similar, differentiation is difficult. There are a few criteria that can be used to determine the nature of the lesion. Metastatic cancers most often appear in the fat that surrounds the breast parenchyma and are most often near the midline or in the fatty tail. Second primary cancers, in contrast, occur in the breast tissue, most often in the upper outer quadrant. Metastatic cancers tend to be multiple and grow in an expansile fashion, while primary ones tend to be single and have a stellate, crablike pattern. If the nuclear grade of the lesion in the second breast is distinctly greater than in the first breast, then the cancer is considered to be primary. The lesion in the second breast is judged to be primary if foci consistent with a site of origin are present or if the breast tissue shows pronounced epithelial hyperplasia. In primary tumors, contiguous in situ carcinoma is the rule. An exception is medullary carcinoma, around which in situ changes are not common. If the cancer in the second breast appears more than five years later than in the first breast and there is no other evidence of metastasis, it is considered to be a primary.

The question that remains unanswered is what to do about the second breast. Should it simply be followed by careful periodic physical examinations alone or in combination with diagnostic aids such as mammography, xerography, and thermography, or should it be randomly biopsied or prophylactically removed? The best approach would seem to be a combination of these various modalities. Random biopsy of the opposite breast is advisable as part of primary therapy for presymptomatic (Stage 0) and Stage 1 and 2 cancers in all patients except the elderly or those with severe constitutional disease. If a second cancer is found, appropriate therapy should be undertaken. If no cancer is found, the patient should be followed carefully by rigorous, periodic physical examination and by diagnostic aids, unless she is in the high risk group for the development of cancer in the second breast, in which case a delayed prophylactic simple mastectomy is advised.

The incidence of cancer in the second breast is not high enough to warrant the routine use of prophylactic contralateral simple mastectomy in all patients. To adopt such a practice would result in many unnecessary operations and add little to the survival rates. I recommend the procedure only in a specific group of patients who have a high risk for developing cancer in the remaining breast. Simultaneous removal of the second breast is also not advisable, since it is emotionally upsetting and precludes proper evaluation as to whether the patient is in the high risk group.

It is true that some patients are adamant in their refusal to have anything done about their second breasts. Many of my patients, however, about three to six months after initial surgery, spontaneously express concern about their second breasts. They are worried about pain, nodularities, and irregularities and the possibility of developing cancer. They often complain of the lack of symmetry and the difficulty of matching the remaining breast with a good prosthesis. If such a patient is in the high risk group, I discuss with her the advantages of prophylactic removal of her second breast, emphasizing that this procedure would be of much less magnitude than her first, that the incision would be transverse and would not show with her bra on, that her muscle would not be disturbed, that she would have excellent function and no edema, and that a reconstruction could be done at a later date. If she is not a high risk patient or if she refuses surgery, I simply tell her that I will follow the other breast very carefully.

The patients I have performed delayed prophylactic simple mastectomy on have had an increase rather than a decrease in mental and physical comfort. Fear of developing cancer in the remaining breast is removed, symmetry is restored. The patient no longer feels unbalanced and has much greater ease in dressing, bathing, and movements. Only a few patients have expressed regret over the loss of the second breast and most have been pleased with the results. If the first breast has been removed by a modified radical mastectomy, reconstruction using silicone implants can be done, offering a good cosmetic result.

To date I have performed delayed prophylactic simple (complete) contralateral mastectomy in only 97 patients, all of whom were in the high risk group. The remaining breast in each case was asymptomatic, without clinical or mammographic evidence of cancer. Seventeen unsuspected cancers were found, an incidence of 17.5%. Five were infiltrating and 12 were noninfiltrating. In addition, 15 specimens showed precancerous mastopathy (15.5%). Of 63 patients followed for over five years, 3 have died, a survival rate of 95.3%. This figure does not support the theory that the trauma entailed in the removal of the second breast might exacerbate carcinogenic developments which might have been reversed or progressed more slowly without this added trauma.

DR. LESTER: I expect there are many questions from the audience. If the panel participants want to argue among themselves, that, too, is permitted.

QUESTION: Dr. Hutter, I was amazed at the diagram you showed with the multiple foci in the one breast. Is this not a perfect argument against a simplified procedure such as lumpectomy?

DR. HUTTER: Some people have wanted to use it that way, but I do not think it is. We know multiplicity is frequent, but we really do not have specific data to tell us its significance. In Hayward's study, there was no lack of control of the disease in the breast when they did less than a mastectomy and followed it by radiation. This is where we have to keep our eyes open. We are gathering data, but have not totally assessed its significance.

DR. LESTER: Dr. Leis, would you like to comment on that question?

DR. LEIS: This is a tricky point. You cannot argue with the work of Gallager and Martin, who have shown that there is a high percentage of multicentricity, nor can you argue with the work that Dr. Hutter has shown or with Dr. Egan. Not all breast cancers are multicentric, of course, but who has the nerve to say whether or not in a specific patient the cancer is multicentric? What is the rationale of removing part of the breast, leaving the woman with a smaller, deformed breast, rather than doing a total mastectomy and allowing her to have a plastic reconstruction?

DR. URBAN: I would like to comment on the data of Hayward and Atkins, which showed a good 10 year salvage in Stage 1 breast cancer treated by lumpectomy and 2900 rads to the breast. Statements have been made that this therapy will not result in radiation-induced cancers, but nobody knows. The data from Hiroshima indicate otherwise. More than a few of the people who survived the atomic bomb developed leukemias soon thereafter. Fifteen or 20 years later, a significant number of women developed breast cancer. If they were exposed to 90 rads, the incidence was double the expected rate and for every additional 40 rads the increment was twofold. I think we may be in for some disappointing results 15 or 20 years from now in the patients who are being treated by lumpectomy with aggressive radiotherapy.

DR. LESTER: I am glad you raised that point. Dr. Powers on the previous panel, suggested that chronic low dose radiation was carcinogenic, but high dose acute radiation not. The results in breast cancer, and a number of other lesions as well, indicate that high dose acute radiation can also be carcinogenic under varying circumstances. I believe the time is up and we must conclude this panel.

Low Dose Mammography

HAROLD J. ISARD, M.D.
ALAN S. BAKER, M.S.

Approximately a decade ago, Dr. Richard Chamberlain delivered the
annual oration at the Philadelphia Roentgen Ray Society. It was enti-
tled "The Thrifty Use of Radiation," and emphasized the need to obtain a maximum of diagnostic information with the least radiation exposure
to the patient.

There has been a report by MacKenzie indicating an increased incidence
of breast cancer among women who had had multiple fluoroscopic examinations during treatment for pulmonary tuberculosis. A group of women
treated with x-rays for acute postpartum mastitis was found to have a greater
incidence of breast cancer than a similar control group, and it has been
reported that Japanese women exposed during the bombing of Hiroshima
and Nagasaki also had a greater incidence. While the radiation exposure
resulting from diagnostic mammography is insignificant by comparison, it is
nevertheless incumbent on us to be thrifty with radiation.

About 15 years ago we made some attempts to lower the mammographic
radiation dose by utilizing a screen system, but the results were unsatisfactory. Our interest was rekindled in 1970 by the report of Price and Butler
that a significant dose reduction could be achieved by the use of nonscreen
film and a single screen vacuum packed in a thin polyethylene envelope.
This suggested the possibility of further reduction in radiation by utilizing
single emulsion film and an intensifying screen. With the advice and encour-
agement of the Photo Products Department of the DuPont Company, a
cooperative study was initiated. DuPont experimented with a variety of film
and screens and we evaluated the products. After approximately a year and
a half, we were both satisfied that we had found a system that provided high
quality images at a significant reduction in patient exposure. Serendipi-

193

tously, there was improvement in the contrast of the soft tissue structures of the breast as compared to conventional mammographic techniques. The system consists of a single emulsion film and a high definition screen, vacuum packed in a light-proof polyethylene bag.

Accurate radiographic interpretation depends in large measure on the quality of the image. Visibility of detail is affected by contrast, sharpness, and the underlying mottle inherent in radiographs. The use of a screen system with maximal contact between film and screen enhances contrast, which is important in the examination of soft tissues with low inherent contrast. Sharpness is also enhanced by the close contact of film and screen and by elimination of the crossover exposure that is characteristic of double emulsion film.

Film grain and screen structure contribute to radiographic mottle or "noise," but more important is the factor of quantum mottle, the result of fluctuations in the distribution of the x-ray quanta absorbed by the screen. There must be sufficient x-ray quanta to minimize such fluctuations and produce uniform film blackening. If the film used is too fast, an image can be obtained with few quanta, but there will be objectionable mottle.

Comparison of the single emulsion film-screen system with nonscreen film showed that high quality radiographs could be obtained with a marked reduction in radiographic exposure (Figures 1 and 2). Soft tissue contrast was accentuated in films made by the Einstein system and microcalcifications were just as clearly visualized. The results also compared well with those of xeromammography (Figure 3).

Surface radiation doses were recorded using lithium fluoride discs placed directly on the patients' breasts. A polystyrene phantom $25 \times 25 \times 5$ cm was used for verification. Three commercially available mammographic units were tested. The phantom, with a lithium fluoride disc on its surface, was positioned as for a mammographic study and series of exposures corresponding to various techniques were made. The results were tabulated and verified with a Capintec 192 electrometer with an 0.6 cc ionization chamber. The electrometer and chamber are traceable to a National Bureau of Standards certification. The data thus collected are shown in Figure 4.

Each of the units contains a molybdenum target tube, and it is apparent that the absorbed dose is comparable for all three units. The MAS variation required for adequate exposures reflects the geometric differences in the three units. The AEMC technique gave an absorbed dose of approximately 1.5 to 2.0 rads for an average breast as compared to 13.0 to 14.0 rads when Eastman Kodak AA film was the recording material. Ascribing unity to the Einstein system, the relative MAS's required at 30 kV for satisfactory exposures are shown in Table 1.

Table 2 lists the advantages and disadvantages of the film-screen system compared to nonscreen film.

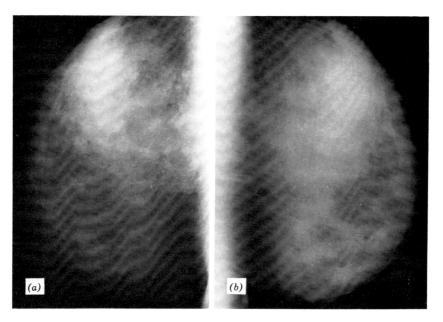

Figure 1. Comparable lateral views of the breast. *(a)* Film-screen combination; *(b)* Kodak AA film. Note the enhanced contrast and better definition of microcalcifications.

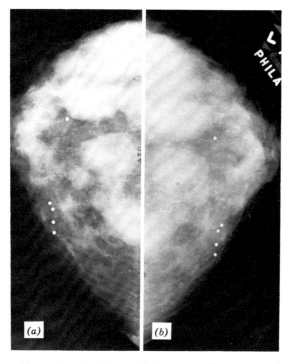

Figure 2. Comparable craniocaudad views of the breast. *(a)* Film-screen combination; *(b)* Kodak AA film. Contrast is enhanced and nodular masses better defined.

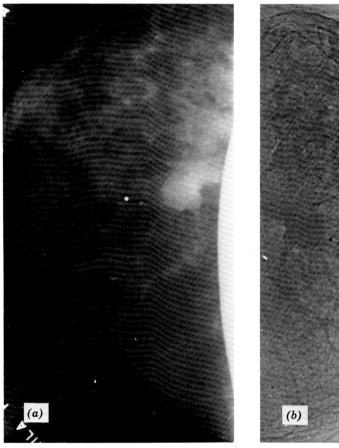
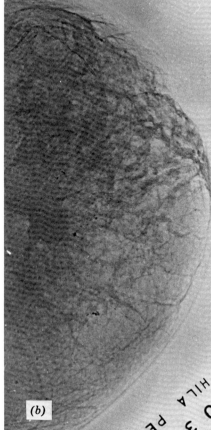

Figure 3. *(a)* Low dose film; *(b)* Xerox image of malignant mass.

Table 1   Relative MAS

Single emulsion film and intensifying screen	**1.0**
Nonscreen film—medical (OSRAY-M)	**2.4**
Nonscreen film—industrial (Kodak AA)	**8.0**

In summary, by combining a single emulsion film with a high definition screen, mammograms of excellent quality are obtained with a significant reduction in radiation dose.

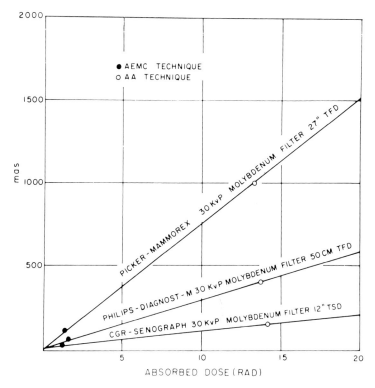

Figure 4. Measured surface radiation dose for three different mammographic techniques.

Table 2

	Advantages	Disadvantages
Special film and screen combination [a]	Low patient dose Enhanced contrast Rapid automatic processing Short exposure time Less motion unsharpness	Potential screen artifacts Minimal mottle
Nonscreen film (industrial type)	Grainless image	High patient dose Hand or prolonged automatic processing Long exposure time Motion unsharpness Overheat x-ray tube

[a] DuPont single emulsion film and single high definition screen.

Comparison Study of Xeromammography and Lo-dose Mammography

RUTH E. SNYDER, M.D.
ROBERTA L.A. KIRCH, M.D.

Over the years, mammography techniques have continued to evolve. In 1970 Memorial Hospital began to use the Senograph with hand developed AA film. This was a great improvement over the tungsten target as far as contrast and detail were concerned, although the radiation dose was still relatively high. For one year, from 1972 to 1973, xeroradiography alone was employed for mammography. There were many technical difficulties and many errors in diagnosis. After Isard demonstrated Lo-dose film at the Mammographic Conference at San Diego in 1973, it was decided to begin a dual study using both Lo-dose and xeroradiography on each patient.

Two experienced examiners participated, reading independently. One read only films (RES) and the other only xeroradiograms (RLAK). Quality was listed as good, adequate, or poor. Diagnosis was recorded as (a) no lesion; (b) benign lesion; (c) significant lesion (probably benign); (d) probably malignant; and (e) definitely malignant. The xerograms and mammograms were reviewed together when there was a discrepancy in diagnosis between the two readers or an error was discovered after biopsy.

Using the Senograph, the factors for xeroradiography were 40 kV, 30 MAS, and 0.5 mm aluminum filtration. For film mammography 30 kV, 40 MAS, and 0.03 mm molybdenum filtration was used. The average exposure dose was approximately 1 rad for film and 3.5 rads for xeroradiography.

199

The quality judgment for the two examinations was about the same; 63% of the mammography studies and 61% of the xeroradiograms were rated as good, 32% of the mammograms and 33% of xeroradiograms adequate, and 5% of mammograms and 6% of the xerograms poor. The standards for judging the quality of mammograms were higher than for xeroradiograms because the previous technique with hand developed film served as a reference. With the Lo-dose film, dirty screens were occasionally a problem. Poor processing also interfered significantly with quality and, therefore, a separate processor used only for mammography has now been installed. Serious artifacts appeared to be inherent in the xeroradiographic system. It was difficult to buy defect free plates; latent or residual images from previous studies, powder deficiency spots, and pressure marks were frequent. A high "downtime" for servicing was also found and over 100 patients had to be excluded from this dual study because the Xerox equipment was not functional. However, overall quality was judged to be at least acceptable in 94–95% of the cases for both techniques.

During the period of 13 months included in this study 1473 patients were examined. This represents 2631 breasts. Biopsies were performed on 209 breasts of 169 patients. Of these, 161 were benign and 48 malignant. Of the benign cases biopsied, 86% of the mammograms and 87% of the xerograms were correctly diagnosed as benign. Twenty-one mammograms and 18 xeroradiograms were over-called. One case eventually proved to be malignant. There were a few instances in which the interpretation was probably malignant in which the biopsy showed atypical hyperplasia, a lesion that is considered to be premalignant. A few cases were sclerosing adenosis which is known to mimic cancer.

Of the 48 patients with cancer, the Lo-dose film study missed four cases and xeroradiogram seven cases. One of the cases missed by both methods was lobular carcinoma in situ. Most of the other cancers could not be identified even in retrospect. The cases missed by xeroradiography alone were usually at the margin of the plate, in the subareolar region or medial in position. Seven malignancies were called "probably benign" by each method. This does not mean that they were not demonstrated but that the abnormality was coded as "probably benign." In such a case, we suggest biopsy, correlation with clinical findings, or reexamination after a short period. The accuracy rate for a *specific* diagnosis of cancer was 77% for Lo-dose film mammography and 64% for xeroradiography. However, the detection rate for a significant abnormality was 91% for Lo-dose film mammography and 86% for xeroradiography. The difference is probably too small to be statistically valid with so few cases.

In 30 months of hospital experience with xeroradiography and 15 months of use of Lo-dose films in hospital and office practice, approximately 3000 xeroradiographic studies and 11,000 Lo-dose examinations have been performed. Both systems are superior to film study using tungsten target and have a relatively high accuracy rate. A compilation of advantages and disadvantages of each system is given in Tables 1 and 2.

Table 1   Advantages

Xeroradiography	Lo-dose Mammography
High accuracy	High accuracy
Roomlight viewing	Low radiation
Less eye fatigue and pleasing appearance	Excellent detail
Easily reproduced for publication	Short exposure minimizes motion
Daylight processing	Delayed or remote processing possible
90 seconds processing	Very reliable equipment
	Coned views possible
	Can be phototimed
	90 seconds processing
	Better technician acceptance

Table 2   Disadvantages

Xeroradiography	Lo-dose Mammography
Relatively higher radiation dose for patient	Artifacts due to dirty screens or processor
Masses not well seen near margins, chest wall, in medial position, or in subareolar region	Requires vacuum packing
Serious artifacts appear to be inherent in the system: Powder deficiency spots (PDS), plate defects, toner robbing, halos around calcifications, roller marks, latent images, and plates sensitive to pressure	Requires darkroom processing
High *maintenance* downtime	
High cost (minimum $650 per month plus supplies and plates)	
Plates must be charged, used, and processed without delays	
Requires additional floor space in examination room.	
45 minutes initial warm-up for system	

The xeroradiograms have no more exposure latitude than the Lo-dose film. Masses are not well seen near the chest wall and in the subareolar region or in the medial half of the breast unless a lateral-medial film is taken. The plates must be charged, used, and processed without delay to avoid deterio-

ration of the image. It is also not possible to do cone or pressure views. The rental charges and supplies constitute an additional expense.

The short exposure time for Lo-dose film has been found to minimize motion and it also appears to have extended the tube life of the Senograph. The technicians find the Lo-dose film technique to be easy and fast. The only difficulty is that the screens and processor must be kept meticulously clean.

In summary, the disadvantages of xeroradiography have been sufficiently serious that Memorial Hospital has discontinued its use. The convincing advantages of Lo-dose mammography have been the lower radiation dose to the patient, the accuracy, the economy, and the reliability when compared with xeroradiography.

Programmed Instruction in Mammographic Interpretation

FRANKLIN S. ALCORN, M.D.

Errors in diagnostic radiology derive not so much from technical imperfections in films as from constant and often unsuitable responses on the part of film readers to the information presented to them. Utilizing experience gained in previous attempts to train nonphysician personnel to scan mammographic films, a system of modified program learning was developed.

The theoretical basis of programmed instruction lies in the stimulus-response theory developed by Edward Thorndike and later modified by Skinner and others. These early investigators contributed evidence suggesting that the student, in the presence of a stimulus, would make responses intended to move him beyond obstacles to his goal. As knowledge of programmed learning increased, the concept of reinforcement or "feedback" was introduced in 1954. This feedback of information enabled the learner to recognize the correctness of his response to the learning stimulus. If the response is correct and adequate, the psychological effect is to "reward" the response and thus enhance the learning mechanism (Figure 1). Although not originally designed with the intention that the student would use programmed material for initial coverage of a subject, it became apparent that the concept of presenting material in small individual steps and making use of the law of immediacy as well as correctness of responses was extremely valuable in industrial training.

This method at first was not applied to any great extent to the teaching of

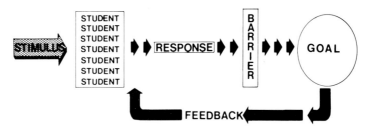

Figure 1   Diagrammatic representation of the sequence of events in the learning process.

academic subjects, but Quakenbush noted that by 1961 there were more than 30 published research studies on the use of programmed instruction, and that the effectiveness of the method was confirmed by actual classroom utilization.

Developing a strict Skinnerian program for a course is time consuming and difficult, often requiring considerable consultation with a programming expert. We might ask whether this additional work is necessary or helpful in teaching scientific and medical subjects. There are many studies in the literature comparing the results of programmed teaching with more traditional methods. Most authors agree that it is difficult to test objectively the differences, because there have been few attempts to provide instruction to similar groups of students on identical subject matter prepared for programmed presentation and also by the traditional textbook-lecture method. The advantages of programmed learning, however, may be summarized by saying that students of lower achievement levels have apparently benefited by the programmed approach. The method has a distinct leveling influence. Test scores are generally higher among students using the program. In addition, the programmed approach was apparently preferred by students and teachers. Programmed material enables the student to proceed in small steps, thus covering the material in the laboratory or classroom time. It also makes it easy for the instructor to pinpoint errors, and areas not clearly understood may be rectified by changing a frame in the program.

The disadvantage of programming lies in the failure to achieve cognitive learning. The student is merely required to recognize rather than understand in most programs. This places too much emphasis on passive learning. Many also feel that there is a tendency to condition responses to verbal patterns, which leads to parroting. Others feel that programmed learning does not further the students' skills in clear, effective thought communication. None of these are disadvantages in the teaching of mammographic screening.

Following the principles of Mager and utilizing a format proposed by William J. Tuddenham, the educational objectives for our program were stated. Briefly, these objectives were that the student would learn to conduct a thorough search of the mammogram and to identify abnormal shadows, separating them from the normal background. The student would also learn to evaluate the technical quality of a mammogram, thus enabling him to reject those films not adequate for the detection of vital information. The teaching materials were designed to provide step-by-step directions concerning the diagnostic signs to be identified, and illustrations of each sign, so that its distinctive properties could be recognized among the faint gray shadows that compose the breast stroma.

In the preliminary work, it was apparent that this recognition constituted the most difficult aspect of mammographic screening. There are both physiological and psychological bases for this difficulty. It has been shown that the movement of a distinct border across the retina produces a maximal cortical response in experimental animals. This explains the "arresting" effect on the scanning eye of distinct masses, which, fortunately, constitute most of the important diagnostic signs of malignant neoplasms. Indistinct shadows produce less retinal excitation. Unless there is a heightened expectation on the part of the observer, they will probably be overlooked. This, in all likelihood, explains the failure to perceive certain important diagnostic signs in the mammograms.

Tuddenham, in his summary of the physiologic and psychologic aspects of perception, describes the close relationship of perception to contrast and definition. Ambiguous and photographically inconspicuous shadows are not perceived unless there is a substantial degree of "recognition" on the part of the observer. The perception of such shadows depends on an innate search for "meaning." This search is influenced by past experience in the development of a high degree of expectation on the part of the observer. The perceived "whole" is constructed by the observer from his own store of memories. On these, he is able to construct a plausible explanation for partial or fragmentary diagnostic signs. This is particularly important in the detection of faint masses.

The development of the flow chart was difficult, but its flexibility makes it more appropriate to reading mammographic analysis than a strict Skinnerian program. The flow chart, in effect, becomes a primary teaching device. The objectives specified for student mammographic scanners are purposely relatively simple. It is required only that they learn to detect diagnostically critical roentgen shadows. It is not necessary to discriminate between abnormal shadows of differing diagnostic values or to arrive at specific diagnostic possibilities. This makes a simple linear type of flow sheet possible. The flow chart offers a direct approach to teaching the student. It builds up the memory store of diagnostic signs so that they can be sorted out from the miasm of ambiguous gray shadows that constitutes a mammogram (Figure 2).

It was determined during the development of the learning tree that there

Using a magnifying lens, do you see 3 or more calcifications in the ductal
complex of the breast?

┌──────── Yes   No ──────────▶

Are the calcifications clustered or localized?

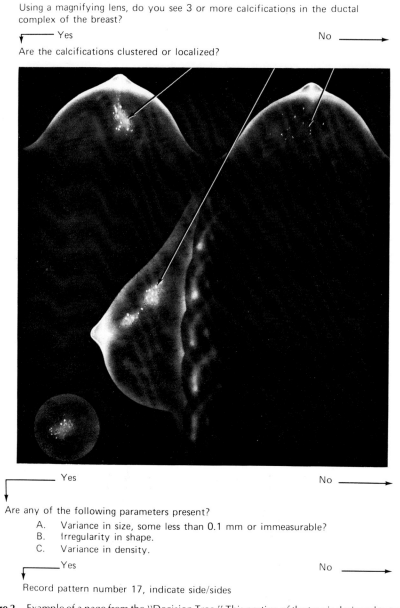

┌──────── Yes   No ──────────▶
│
▼

Are any of the following parameters present?

    A.   Variance in size, some less than 0.1 mm or immeasurable?
    B.   Irregularity in shape.
    C.   Variance in density.

┌──────── Yes   No ──────────▶
│
▼

Record pattern number 17, indicate side/sides

Figure 2 Example of a page from the "Decision Tree." This portion of the tree is designed to teach
the scanner to search carefully for small calcifications.

are 27 separate diagnostic criteria or patterns for the mammographic
identification of malignant disease. A number of these patterns, that is,
nonsmooth bordered masses with calcification, small clusters of calcification
alone, and irregular masses, are highly specific. Others, for example, skin

changes, increased vascularity, and altered trabeculae, are indicators of malignancy to a lesser extent.

Reordering of these diagnostic signs into graded and weighted lists lends itself to the statistical estimation or probability diagnosis of malignancy. Preliminary work has been done by Ackerman et al. utilizing 36 radiographic properties. A semiquantitative question sheet was designed to provide numerical measures of the sizes, distribution, and descriptions of lesions (Figure 3). The list was designed to simulate the decision procedure of a radiologist.

In order to accomplish this, the questions were divided into three parts. The first was a comparison between right and left breast mammograms, identifying normal anatomy. This enabled the observer to note differences between the two sides, since the breasts in comparable views are almost mirror images in a given individual. Areas of difference were labeled as suspicious. In part two, the radiologist assigned descriptors for each suspicious area and described the abnormalities in detail expressing the differences in quantitative terms. Part three covered indications of malignancy removed from the suspicious areas. These were identified and suitably described.

A questionnaire was then devised from the three parts. The first 12

CLASSIFICATION OF BREAST TUMORS

1. Do you see calcifications in or about the suspicious area or near it?
   1. None
   2. In it, central
   3. In it, peripheral
   4. In it, evenly distributed
   5. In it and about it
   6. Near it

2. Do you see calcifications? (Exclude vascular calcifications).
   1. No
   2. Yes I do
   3. I think I do
   4. I think I don't
   (If answer is no, skip to question #27)

3. Count the number of calcifications

4. Are these clusters?
   1. Very densely packed-some calcifications touching
   2. In a cluster
   3. Seem to be slightly grouped
   4. Randomly distributed

5. Calcification shape.
   1. Round to ovoid
   2. Elongated rods
   3. Ring
   4. Varied shape, i.e., amorphous
   5. Punctate-too small to describe
   6. Irregular
   7. Answers 1 and 2
   8. Answers 3 and 4
   9. Answers 5 and 6

7. Do you see variability of density among the calcifications?
   1. No
   2. Yes
   3. Not sure

8. Calcification size.
   1. Can barely see with magnifying glass
   2. .5 mm to .75 mm diameter
   3. .75 mm to 1.5 mm diameter
   4. 2.0 mm to 2.5 mm diameter
   5. 2.5 mm to greater diameter
   6. Answers 2 and 3
   7. Answers 4 and 5
   8. Answers 1 and 2
   9. Answers 3 and 4

Figure 3 A section from the question sheet that was devised to provide information on the size, shape, and distribution of calcifications.

questions provided a description of normal anatomy, the next 8 dealt with a description of each suspicious area, and the final 8 covered descriptions of any secondary signs of cancer.

Following the completion of the questionnaire, the properties were ranked according to their estimated importance by the rated sum of two criteria: (a) the expected probability of error (POE) of the individual properties; and (b) the average correlation coefficient (ACC) of properties whose POE values were small. This was done in order to determine if a fraction of the important properties could be used to make decisions equal in quality to decisions made using all the properties (Figure 4).

The validity of the hypothesis was evaluated by utilizing a test set of size and composition comparable to the training set. It was found that a false

Computer-ordered Properties in Descending Order of Importance

Property number	Property description
16	Mass diameter
2	Percentage peripheral fat
15	Mass border
12	No. suspicious areas
34	No. axillary massess
14	Mass smoothness
27	Nipple inversion
4	Mottled pattern presence
13	Mass density
9	Duct beadiness
28	Vein pattern
22	No. calcifications
18	Halo
31	Skin retraction
29	Vein size ratio
10	No. poorly defined masses
5	Percentage mottling
20	Presence of mass calcifications
11	No. well-defined masses
36	Maximum axillary node diameter
17	Mass location
3	Percentage internal glandular fat
33	Straightened thickened trabeculae
32	Subareolar thickening
6	Number ductal patterns
1	Fat margin border
35	Average node diameter
25	Calcification density
19	Adjacent mass trabeculations
7	Duct path description
26	Calcification size
30	Skin thickness
8	Duct size
21	Calcification presence
24	Calcification shape
23	Calcification clusters

Figure 4 List of the 36 properties studied, in descending order of importance.

positive rate of 55% was obtained. There were no false negatives. Most of the errors made by this method were in cases in which the radiologist had not offered a definitive diagnosis.

Although it is improper to extrapolate from such a small data base, it is believed that this approach, utilizing the diagnostic parameters described, when combined with related information obtained by history and physical examination, should provide a probability diagnosis of malignancy with a reasonable degree of accuracy.

A modified program learning approach is a convenient and rapid method of familiarizing students with the diagnostic signs of malignant neoplasms. The pattern-recognition approach lends itself to computer analysis. In the future, combining mammographic evidence with information obtained from history and physical examination may enable us to derive a probability diagnosis for cancer of the breast.

Automation of Thermographic Screening

ALFONSO ZERMENO, Ph.D.

In applying thermography to mass screening for breast cancer, there are many techniques that can be employed to help ease the burden on technicians and thereby allow more patients to be screened per day. Over the last three years, we have developed an approach to this problem that encompasses a total thermographic system rather than a thermographic scanner alone. This system makes use of a remote controlled positioner for the patient, a scan-rate converter to present the thermographic image at conventional television rates, a video disc or video tape recorder for storage of images, a photographic recorder and processor that produces images mounted on computer data cards, and a central console to integrate the manipulation of these various components.

In developing this concept, it was also necessary to consider room design. Since the thermographic procedure requires precooling of the patient, two or three cooling booths are necessary. Use of a split system, in which the scanning mechanism is packaged separately from the control console, allows more patient privacy, since a screen or room divider may be placed between the operator and the patient. This arrangement and the increased privacy it affords have been found to produce increased patient acceptance by volunteer subjects such as those encountered in mass screening.

In our initial study of thermographic screening, it was found that the most troublesome and time consuming parts of the examination were patient positioning, manipulation of the scanner controls, and obtaining proper focus.

To solve the first of these problems, a conventional secretarial-type swivel chair was modified by the addition of a small motor with remote controls to turn the patient from the anteroposterior to the oblique position.

To facilitate the movement of the scanner, both for focusing and for placing the patient within the center of the field of view, we have modified the Hercules tripod by adding small direct current motors on the various drives. The use of these motors allows us now to manipulate remotely the position of the scanner in three directions.

The chief difficulty in obtaining proper focus is that the modern thermographic scanners have relatively slow frame rates, that is, two or three seconds per frame. Since the thermal scan takes approximately two seconds, it is necessary to make a complete scan, and, if the patient is not in focus, wait an additional two seconds to evaluate the effect of prior adjustments.

Our solution to this problem was the development of a dual ended laser that produces two converging beams of light that strike the patient's chest wall when placed at a predetermined distance of two feet. The scanner-to-patient distance is varied until the two beams converge on the chest wall at the predetermined focal distance.

A remote control console subsequently developed contains joy sticks that control the focal adjustment, the adjustment of the scanner position, and the rotation of the patient chair. A monitor allows the technician to view the patient on closed circuit television. In addition, two television monitors are employed to display the thermal image both in black hot and white hot modes.

To these components of the system, we have now added a modified camera-processor manufactured by the 3M Corporation. This device has been used for many years in industry for microfilming of documents and reprints. In conjunction with design engineers of the 3M Corporation, the machine was adapted to thermography. Interfacing the camera-processor to the thermographic scanner entailed the installation of three television monitors within the device. The three monitors, displaying the stored thermal images, are adjusted to different contrast and brightness settings. A photograph of the three monitors yields three thermal images of the patient effectively at three different thermal settings. In practice, the anteroposterior and right and left oblique views are exposed on a single film chip resulting in a total of nine thermal images per aperture card. After the third exposure, the card is automatically translated into the processor for development and is available for viewing within 45 seconds.

Of the various photographic systems available for thermography today, the Polaroid camera has the advantage of presenting a thermal image within 20 seconds of exposure. The major disadvantage of the Polaroid technique lies in its cost. Seventy millimeter roll film has been employed in a number of installations with a significant saving in cost. Its major disadvantage is the inaccessibility of the image until development of the entire roll. Due to the

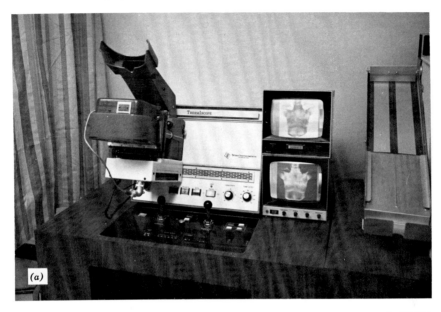

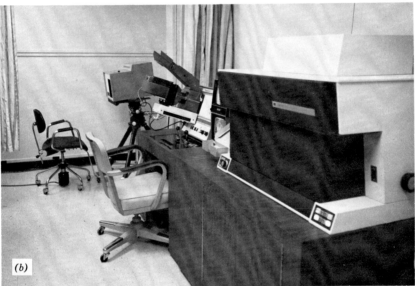

Figure 1. *(a)* The remote control console. At the right are the television screens displaying the thermographic image. *(b)* The four elements of the automated system. From the left, the motorized patient chair, the scanner, the console and the camera-processor.

uncertainty encountered in using 70 mm roll film, users must often make multiple exposures at various machine settings to insure the acquisition of at least one diagnostic image.

With the thermographic system as we have designed it, images are available immediately. The estimated cost of the aperture card, including the cost of chemicals, is about 10 cents. This represents a significant reduction in operating cost in comparison to either the Polaroid or 70 mm film system. In addition, one can store some 80,000 cards in a conventional data card cabinet. The aperture card as designed by 3M has 53 columns available for keypunching of pertinent patient information.

The complete system is now undergoing critical evaluation. It is hoped that data on the feasibility of this approach to mass screening will soon be available. At present, use of this system has enabled us to process some 80 to 90 patients per day with one technician operating the machine.

The Problem of the Isolated Positive Thermogram

GERALD D. DODD, M.D.

The major difficulty with the use of thermography as a screening modality is the frequency of the so-called false positive. If one is concerned with cancer only, a false positive is a positive thermogram in an individual who has no clinical or mammographic evidence of cancer. If, on the other hand, we include all disease of the breast, a false positive is something entirely different. In this sense, few false positives are found. Usually a strongly positive thermogram indicates there is an abnormality in the breast. It does not tell what the abnormality is. It merely means that for some reason there is accelerated metabolic activity in the breast.

In a summary of the world's literature on thermography, the true positive rate was found to be 86%, and the false negative rate was 14%. More important, the so-called false positive rate varied between 15 and 20%.

Many entities have been incriminated as causing positive thermograms. The list covers the spectrum of the pathologic processes that can occur in the breast. Anything that goes wrong in the breast is capable of causing a positive thermogram. In a selected group from our institution, patients who had complaints or abnormalities referable to the breast, the "false positive" rate was 40.4%. This emphasizes my point. The lack of specificity of thermography is reflected in symptomatic patients. It is in the general population of women without complaints that the 15 or 20% false positive rate applies.

How can one know that a lesion found by mammography or biopsy is actually the cause of the positive thermogram? One patient we studied had a definitely abnormal thermogram. Her mammograms showed an asymmetrical density in the upper outer quadrant of the breast. Yet on the thermogram the abnormality lay in the areolar area. She turned out to have a noninvasive intraductal carcinoma in the subareolar region. The prominence seen mammographically was due to fibrosis. In this instance we had a marker from the mammogram. If we had not had the information on the thermogram we would not have known what to do.

Another case in point is a physician's wife. Her thermogram showed abnormal heat around the areola and venous enlargement. The xeromammogram showed bilateral dense breasts with no specific abnormality. On physical examination there were only vague multiple nodules. In desperation, because the thermogram was persistently positive, a biopsy was done. It showed small duct hyperplasia and periductal collagenosis, both changes that may be associated with cancer of the breast. We have followed this patient since 1969, but she has not developed clinical cancer. The thermogram has waxed and waned. We know that cancers show cyclic activity, certainly over a period of 24 hours or so, and probably over periods of months. Short of removing this patient's breast prophylactically, there is no solution.

What is the significance of a persistently positive thermogram in an individual in whom we cannot find any other abnormality? I believe these patients should be regarded as being at risk. An example was a woman 49 years old who had a strongly positive thermogram on the right side when first examined in 1964. The mammogram at that time showed fibrocystic disease. There were no changes suggesting cancer. Fourteen months later, the thermogram was still positive but now the mammogram showed tiny calcifications in the medial upper quadrant. She had an invasive carcinoma 2 or 3 mm in diameter.

Another case in point was a woman who came as the result of a survey procedure. She had a history of fibrocystic disease and a suspicious thermogram. There were no significant findings clinically, and the mammogram showed only bilateral dense breasts. There was a small, isolated calcification. She came back eight months later. The breasts looked the same, but the pattern of the thermogram had changed. There was exaggeration of the venous pattern bilaterally, more pronounced on the left. Physical examination remained the same, as did the mammogram. The next examination was 28 months after the first study. The thermogram showed pronounced engorgement on the left and a prominent venous pattern on the right side. At this time, physical examination showed a 1 cm superficial mass in the left breast that had not been there previously. There were no abnormalities on the right. The mammogram of the left side showed nothing except dense breast. On the right, however, there was an increase in the calcifications first noted two years before. This patient proved to have bilateral carcinoma. A mass appeared on the left 28 months after her first positive thermogram. On the right, carcinoma was manifested only by calcification and no mass, either at the time of surgery or on the mammogram. There was, in this patient, an early indication from the thermogram that an abnormality was present, but we were unable to do anything but follow her until substantiating evidence appeared.

We have recently surveyed 4700 patients by thermography, and of these 635 have had abnormal thermograms for which there is no explanation. That is approximately 13.5%. Our follow-up is incomplete, but of that group of 635, 32, or 5%, of the "false positives" have subsequently developed carcinoma in the breast that was originally incriminated.

I would like to give you a lot of facts and figures like these, but I cannot do it. Thermography is not an examination that depends on morphology as does the mammogram. It is a dynamic abnormality that is subject to change from hour to hour, and day to day, and precisely how much and to what degree we do not know. I wish I could tell you how many of these patients with false positives will eventually get cancer, but I cannot.

Despite the fact that thermography has been around for 10 to 12 years, the recent changes in instrumentation and knowledge largely vitiate the results published in the past. We are only now embarking on a meaningful investigation of the technique. In this sense, I think its widespread use is premature. I heartily endorse the investigation of thermography in the screening centers, and hope that the information that is derived therefrom will put thermography into its proper perspective.

Bibliographic References

Ackerman, L. V., Mucciardi, A. N., Gose, Earl E., and Alcorn, F. S.: Classification of benign and malignant breast tumors on the basis of 36 radiographic properties. *Cancer,* **31:**342–352, 1973.

Ackerman, L. V.: An evaluation of the treatment of cancer of the breast at the University of Edinburgh (Scotland) under the direction of Dr. Robert McWhirter. *Cancer,* **8:**883, 1955.

Ackerman, L. V., and Del Regato, J. A.: *Cancer: Diagnosis, Treatment and Prognosis.* 4th edition. St. Louis, Missouri, C. V. Mosby Co., 1970.

Alcorn, F. S., O'Donnell, E., and Ackerman, L. V.: The protocol and results of training nonradiologists to scan mammograms. *Radiology,* **99:**523–529, 1971.

Alcorn, F. S., and O'Donnell, E.: Mammography screeners—Modified program learning for nonradiologic personnel. *Radiology,* **90:**336–368, 1968.

Alcorn, F. S., and O'Donnell, E.: The training of nonphysician personnel for use in a mammography program. *Cancer,* **23:**879–883, 1969.

Anderson, D. E.: A genetic study of human breast cancer. *Journal of the National Cancer Institute,* **48:**1029–1034, 1972.

Anderson, D. E.: Some characteristics of familial breast cancer. *Cancer,* **28:**1500–1504, 1971.

Anderson, D. E.: Genetic study of breast cancer: Identification of a high-risk group. *Cancer,* in press.

Axel, R., Schlom, J., and Spiegelman, S.: Presence in human breast cancer of RNA homologous to mouse mammary tumor virus RNA. *Nature,* **235:**32–36, 1972.

Benfield, J. R., Fingerhut, A. G., and Warner, N. E.: Lobular carcinoma of the breast. *Archives of Surgery,* **99:**129, August 1969.

Bottomley, R. H., Trainer, A. L., and Condit, P. T.: Chromosome studies in a "cancer family." *Cancer,* **28:**519–528, 1971.

Burch, J. C., and Byrd, B. F., Jr.: Effects of long-term administration of estrogen on the occurrence of mammary cancer in women. *Annals of Surgery,* **174:**414–418, 1971.

Burns, B. D., Baron, W., and Pritchart, R.: Physiological excitation of visual cortices in cats' unanesthetized isolated forebrain. *Journal of Neurophysiology,* **25:**165–181, March 1962.

Clark, R. L., Copeland, M. M., Egan, R. L., Gallager, H. S., Lindsay, J. P., Robbins, L. C., and White, E. C.: Reproducibility of the technique of mammography (Egan) for cancer of the breast. *American Journal of Surgery,* **109:**127–133, 1965.

Clemmesen, J.: Statistical studies in the aetiology of malignant neoplasms. I. Review and results. *Acta Pathologica et Microbiologica Scandinavica,* Suppl. **174:**1–543, 1965.

Cooper, T., Randall, W. C., and Hertzman, A. B.: Vascular convection of heat from active muscle to overlying skin. *Journal of Applied Physiology,* **14:**207, 1959.

de Waard, F., Baanders-van Halewijn, E. A., and Huizinga, J.: The bimodal age distribution of patients with mammary carcinoma: Evidence for the existence of two types of human breast cancer. *Cancer,* **17:**141–151, 1964.

Deterline, W.: *An Introduction to Program Instruction.* New York, N.Y., Prentice-Hall, 1962.

Dodd, G. D., Zermeno, A., Marsh, L., Boyd, D., and Wallace, J. D.: New developments in breast thermography—High spatial resolution. *Cancer,* **24:**121, 1969.

Dodd, G. D., Zermeno, A., Wallace, J. D., and Marsh, L. M.: Breast thermography—The state of the art. *Current Problems in Radiology,* **3:**1–47, 1973.

Egan, R. L.: Mammography, an aid to diagnosis of breast carcinoma. *Journal of the American Medical Association,* **182:**839–843, 1962.

Egan, R. L.: Mammography and diseases of the breast. *CA,* **18:**279, September–October 1968.

Egan, R. L.: Roles of mammography in the early detection of breast cancer. *Cancer,* **24:**1197, December 1969.

Farrow, J. L.: Clinical consideration and treatment of in-situ lobular breast cancer. *American Journal of Roentgenology, Radium Therapy and Nuclear Medicine,* **102:**652, 1968.

Fechner, R. E.: Breast cancer during oral contraceptive therapy. *Cancer,* **26:**1204–1211, 1970.

Fechner, R. E.: The surgical pathology of the reproductive system and breast during oral contraceptive therapy. *Pathology Annual,* **6:**299–319, 1971.

Fink, R., Shapiro, S., and Lewison, J.: The reluctant participant in a breast cancer screening program. *Public Health Reports,* **83:**479–490, 1968.

Fink, R., Shapiro, S., and Roeser, R.: Impact of efforts to increase participation in repetitive screenings for early breast cancer detection. *American Journal of Public Health,* **62:**328–336, 1972.

Finkel, M. P., Biskis, B. O., and Farrell, C.: Osteosarcomas appearing in Syrian hamsters after treatment with extracts of human osteosarcomas. *Proceedings of the National Academy of Sciences,* **60:**1223–1230, 1968.

Foote, F. W., Jr., and Stewart, F. W.: A histological classification of carcinoma of the breast. *Surgery,* **19:**74, 1946.

Ghys, R., *Thermographie Medicale,* Paris, France, Maloine, S.A. 1973, 119 pp.

Gold, R. H., Main, G., Zippin, C. and Annes, G.: Infiltration of mammary carcinoma as an indicator of axillary node metastases. *Cancer,* **29:**35, 1972.

Goldenberg, E. E., Wiegenstein, L., and Mottet, N. K.: Florid breast fibroadenomas in patients taking hormonal oral contraceptives. *American Journal of Clinical Pathology,* **49:**52–59, 1968.

Gray, L. A.: Hormones and pathological lesions of the breast. *Transactions of the Southern Surgical Association,* **81:**247–255, 1970.

Haagensen, C. D.: Family history of breast carcinoma in women predisposed to develop breast carcinoma. *Journal of the National Cancer Institute,* **48:**1025–1027, 1972.

Haddow, Sir Alexander: Presidential Address: IXth International Cancer Congress, Tokyo, 1966.

Herrmann, J. F.: Breast cancer and associated extramammary malignant neoplasms. *American Journal of Surgery,* **124:**620–624, 1972.

Herrman, J. B.: Bilateral breast cancer. *Surgery, Gynecology and Obstetrics,* **136:**771, 1973.

Hertz, R.: The role of steroid hormones in the etiology and pathogenesis of cancer. *American Journal of Obstetrics and Gynecology,* **98:**1013–1019, 1967.

Hutchinson, G. B., and Shapiro, S.: Lead time gained by diagnostic screening for breast cancer. *Journal of the National Cancer Institute,* **41:**665–681, 1968.

Hutter, R. V. P., and Foote, F. W.: Lobular carcinoma in situ. Long term follow-up. *Cancer,* **24:**1081, 1969.

Hutter, R. V. P.: *Breast Carcinoma Monograph.* New York, N.Y., Memorial Hospital for Cancer and Allied Diseases, 1973.

Jaros, B. H.: On comparing programming and other teaching methods. *Journal of Medical Education,* **39**:304–310, March 1964.

Kellermann, G., Shaw, C. R., and Luyten-Kellerman, M.: Aryl hydrocarbon hydroxylase inducibility and bronchogenic carcinoma. *New England Journal of Medicine,* **289**:934–937, 1973.

Lawson, R. N.: Implications of surface temperature in the diagnosis of breast cancer. *Canadian Medical Association Journal,* **75**:309, 1956.

Leis, H. P., Jr., and Pilnik, S.: Nipple discharge. *Hospital Medicine,* **6**:29, November 1970.

Leis, H. P., Jr., Pilnik, S., Dursi, J., and Santoro, E.: Nipple discharge. *International Surgery,* **58**:162, March 1973.

Leis, H. P., Jr., Merscheimer, W. L., Black, M., and DeChabron, A.: The second breast. *New York State Journal of Medicine,* **65**:2460, 1965.

Leis, H. P., Jr.: *Diagnosis and Treatment of Breast Lesions.* Flushing, New York, Medical Examinations Publishing Co., 1970.

Leis, H. P., Jr.: Multidisciplinary approach to the early diagnosis of breast cancer. *International Surgery,* **56**:135, 1971.

Leis, H. P., Jr.: Selective, elective, prophylactic, contralateral mastectomy. *Cancer,* **28**:956, 1971.

Leis, H. P., Jr.: Surgical approach to breast cancer. *New York State Journal of Medicine,* **73**:1992, August 1, 1973.

Leis, H. P., Jr.: Premalignant lesions of the breast. In R. Snyderman, Ed. *Problems of the Female Breast as Related to Neoplasm and Reconstruction.* St. Louis, Missouri, C. V. Mosby Co., 1973.

Lemon, H. M.: Review—Genetic predisposition to carcinoma of the breast: Multiple human genotypes for estrogen-16-alpha-hydroxylase activity in Caucasians. *Journal of Surgical Oncology,* **4**:255–273, 1972.

Lewison, E. F., and Neto, A. S.: Bilateral breast cancer at the Johns Hopkins Hospital. *Cancer,* **28**:1297, 1971.

Li, F. P., and Fraumeni, J. F., Jr.: Soft-tissue sarcomas, breast cancer, and other neoplasms. A familial syndrome? *Annals of International Medicine,* **71**:747–752, 1969.

Lilienfeld, A. M.: The epidemiology of breast cancer. *Cancer Research,* **23**:1503–1513, 1963.

Loeb, L.: Further investigation on the origin of tumors in mice. VI. Internal secretion as a factor in the origin of tumors. *Journal of Medical Research,* **40**:477–496, 1919.

Lynch, H. T., and Krush, A. J.: Carcinoma of the breast and ovary in three families. *Surgery, Gynecology and Obstetrics,* **133**:644–648, 1971.

Lynch, H. T., Krush, A. J., Lemon, H. M., Kaplan, A. R., Condit, P. P., and Bottomley, R. H.: Tumor variation in families with breast cancer. *Journal of the American Medical Association,* **222**:1631–1639, 1972.

Macklin, M. T.: Comparison of the number of breast cancer deaths observed in relatives of breast cancer patients, and the number expected on the basis of mortality rates. *Journal of the National Cancer Institute,* **22**:927–951, 1959.

MacMahon, B., Morrison, A. S., Ackerman, L. V., Lattes, R., Taylor, H. B., and Yuasa, S.: Histologic characteristics of breast cancer in Boston and Tokyo. *International Journal of Cancer,* **11**:338–344, 1973.

Mager, R. H.: *Preparing Instructional Objectives.* Palo Alto, California, Feron Publications, 1962.

McClow, M. V., and Williams, A. C.: Mammographic examinations (4030): Ten-year clinical experience in a community medical center. *Annals of Surgery,* **177**:616–619, May 1973.

Moore, D. H., Charney, J., Kramarsky, B., Lasfargues, E. Y., Sarkar, N. H., Brennan, M. J., Burrows, J. H., Sirsat, S. M., Paymaster, J. C., and Vaidya, A. B.: Search for a human breast cancer virus. *Nature,* **229**:611–614, 1971.

Morton, D. L., Hall, W. T., and Malmgren, R. A.: Human liposarcomas: Tissue cultures containing foci of transformed cells with viral particles. *Science,* **165:**813–815, 1969.

Morton, D. L., and Malmgren, R. A.: Human osteosarcomas: Immunologic evidence suggesting an associated infectious agent. *Science,* **162:**1279–1281, 1968.

Owens, G.: Comparison of programmed instruction with conventional lectures in the teaching of electrocardiography to medical students. *Journal of Medical Education,* **40:**1058–1062, 1965.

Post, R. H.: Breast cancer, lactation, and genetics. *Eugenics Quarterly,* **13:**1–29, 1966.

Potolsky, A. I., Heath, C. W., Jr., Buckley, C. E., III, and Rowlands, D. T., Jr.: Lymphorecticular malignancies and immunologic abnormalities in a sibship. *American Journal of Medicine,* **50:**42–48, 1971.

Quakenbush, J.: How effective are auto-instructional materials and devices? *Transcripts on Education,* Vol. 4, December 1961.

Robbins, G. F., and Berg, J. W.: Bilateral primary breast cancers: A prospective clinicopathological study. *Cancer,* **17:**1501, 1964.

Rogers, J. V., and Powell, R. W.: Mammographic indications for biopsy of clinically normal breasts: Correlations with pathologic findings in 72 cases. *American Journal of Roentgenology, Radiation Therapy and Nuclear Medicine,* **115:**794–800, 1972.

Rosen, P., Snyder, R. E., Urban, J., and Robbins, G.: Correlations of suspicious mammograms and x-rays of breast biopsies during surgery. Results in 60 cases. *Cancer,* **31:**656–659, 1973.

Rosen, P., Snyder, R. E., and Robbins, G.: Specimen radiography for nonpalpable breast lesions found by mammography: Procedures and results. *Cancer,* **34:**2028–2033, December 1974.

Schneck, S. A., and Penn, I.: De novo brain tumors in renal transplant recipients. *Lancet,* **1:**983–986, 1971.

Schoenberg, B. S., Greenberg, R. A., and Eisenberg, H.: Occurrence of certain multiple primary cancers in females. *Journal of the National Cancer Institute,* **43:**15–32, 1969.

Scott, W. G.: Diagnostic radiology. In *Guidelines for Cancer Care.* Chicago, Illinois, American College of Surgeons, 1971.

Shah, J. P., Rosen, P. P., and Robbins, G. F.: Bilateral breast cancer. *Surgery, Gynecology and Obstetrics,* **136:**721, 1973.

Shapiro, S., Strax, P., and Venet, L.: Periodic breast cancer screening in reducing mortality from breast cancer. *Journal of the American Medical Association,* **215:**1777–1785, 1971.

Shapiro, S., Strax, P., Venet, L., and Venet, W.: Changes in 5-year breast cancer mortality in a breast cancer screening program. In *Seventh National Cancer Conference Proceedings.* Philadelphia, J. B. Lippincott Co., 1973, pp. 663–678.

Shapiro, S., Strax, P., Venet, L., and Fink, R.: Periodic breast cancer screening. *Archives of Environmental Health,* **15:**547–553, 1967.

Shapiro, S., Strax, P., and Venet, L.: Periodic breast cancer screening. In *Preventive Medicine—Presymptomatic and Early Diagnosis.* London, England, Sir Isaac Pitman & Sons Ltd., 1968, pp. 203–236.

Skinner, B. F.: The science of learning and the art of teaching. *Harvard Educational Review,* Vol. 24, 1954.

Slack, N. H., Bross, I. D. J., Nemoto, T., and Fisher, B.: Experience with bilateral primary carcinoma of the breast. *Surgery, Gynecology and Obstetrics,* **136:**433, 1973.

Snyder, R.: Mammography and lobular carcinoma in situ. *Surgery, Gynecology and Obstetrics,* **122:**255, 1966.

Snyder, R. E., and Rosen, P.: Radiography of breast specimens. *Cancer,* **28:**1608–1611, 1971.

Strax, P., Venet, L., and Shapiro, S.: Value of mammography in reduction of mortality from breast cancer in mass screening. *American Journal of Roentgenology, Radium Therapy and Nuclear Medicine,* **67:**686, 1973.

Strax, P., Venet, L., Shapiro, S., and Gross, S.: Mammography and clinical examination in mass screening of the breast. *Cancer,* **20:**2184–2188, 1967.

Strax, P., Venet, L., and Shapiro, S.: Mass screening in mammary cancer. *Cancer*, **23**:875–878, 1969.

Taylor, H. B.: Oral contraceptives and pathologic changes in the breast. *Cancer*, **28**:1388–1390, 1971.

Tuddenham, W. J.: The use of logical flow charts as an aid in teaching roentgen diagnosis. *American Journal of Roentgenology, Radium Therapy and Nuclear Medicine*, **102**:797–803, 1968.

Tuddenham, W. J., and Calvert, W. P.: Visual search patterns in roentgen diagnosis. *Radiology*, **76**:225–226, 1961.

Tuddenham, W. J.: Visual problems of roentgen interpretation. *New York State Journal of Medicine*, **60**:1234–1238, 1960.

Urban, J. A.: Bilaterality of cancer of the breast: Biopsy of the opposite breast. *Cancer*, **20**:1867–1870, 1967.

Urban, J. A.: The case against delayed operation for breast cancer. *CA*, **21**:132, 1971.

Urban, J. A.: Bilateral breast cancer. *Cancer*, **24**:1310, 1969.

Venet, L., Strax, P., Venet, W., and Shapiro, S.: Adequacies and inadequacies of breast examinations by physicians. *Cancer*, **24**:1187–1191, 1969.

Venet, L., Strax, P., Venet, W., and Shapiro, S.: Adequacies and inadequacies of breast examinations by physicians in mass screening. *Cancer*, **28**:1546–1551, 1971.

Von Berndt, H., and Landmann, R.: Zwei epidemiologische Typen des Mammakarzinoms. *Archiv fur Geschwulstforschung*, **33**:157–168, 1969.

Walder, B. K., Robertson, M. R., and Jeremy, D.: Skin cancer and immunosuppression. *Lancet*, **2**:1282–1283, 1971.

Wood, D. A.: Tumors of the intestines. In *Atlas of Tumor Pathology*. Washington, D.C., Armed Forces Institute of Pathology, 1967.

Woodworth, M.: The application of program learning to medical technology education. *American Journal of Medical Technology*, **31**:317–330, September 1965.

Index